A pulse-racing new Harle

Sexy Surge

Bachelor brothers in the Big Apple!

To the outside world, siblings and surgeons
Logan and Sam Grant have it all. Born into a vastly
wealthy family and with staggeringly successful
medical careers of their own, they have Manhattan
at their feet. Or do they...?

Their relationships with their family are strained, and
when it comes to finding *the one*, it seems their luck
has truly run out. So for now they're focusing on their
ever-deserving patients and their first love—medicine.
It would take two very special women for the brothers
to allow themselves to be swept up into a whirlwind of
romance again...and they may just have found them!

Logan let ex-wife Harper slip through his fingers
once. He can only wonder if it's fate that's brought
her through the doors of his hospital... Can he win her
back? And does she want to be won...?

Find out in

Manhattan Marriage Reunion by JC Harroway

Burned by love, Sam is plowing his passion
into his work, until his new colleague Lucy charms
her way into his guarded heart in

New York Nights with Mr. Right by Tina Beckett

Both available now!

Dear Reader,

Do you have a passion that drives you? Whether it's your job or a hobby or taking care of your family, is it something that you look forward to each day (or at least most days)?

The hero and heroine of *New York Nights with Mr. Right* are both passionate about the work they do. Lucy works with children doing physical therapy, and Sam helps children with facial trauma or problems with the muscles and nerves of the face. When their specialties overlap and they end up working with each other in the same field, they develop an attraction that can't be denied. Thank you for joining Sam and Lucy as they go on a journey of passion...in more ways than one. And maybe, just maybe, this special couple will find love along the way.

I hope you love reading *New York Nights with Mr. Right* as much as I loved writing it. This couple touched my heart and I hope they touch yours, too.

Love,

Tina Beckett

NEW YORK NIGHTS WITH MR. RIGHT

TINA BECKETT

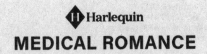

MEDICAL ROMANCE

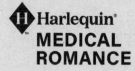

Harlequin®
MEDICAL
ROMANCE

ISBN-13: 978-1-335-94293-7

New York Nights with Mr. Right

Harlequin Enterprises ULC
22 Adelaide St. West, 41st Floor
Toronto, Ontario M5H 4E3, Canada
www.Harlequin.com

Printed in U.S.A.

Recycling programs for this product may not exist in your area.

Three-time Golden Heart® Award finalist **Tina Beckett** learned to pack her suitcases almost before she learned to read. Born to a military family, she has lived in the United States, Puerto Rico, Portugal and Brazil. In addition to traveling, Tina loves to cuddle with her pug, Alex; spend time with her family; and hit the trails on her horse. Learn more about Tina from her website or friend her on Facebook.

Books by Tina Beckett

Harlequin Medical Romance

Alaska Emergency Docs

Reunion with the ER Doctor

Buenos Aires Docs

ER Doc's Miracle Triplets

California Nurses

The Nurse's One-Night Baby

From Wedding Guest to Bride?
A Family Made in Paradise
The Vet, the Pup and the Paramedic
The Surgeon She Could Never Forget
Resisting the Brooding Heart Surgeon
A Daddy for the Midwife's Twins?
Tempting the Off-Limits Nurse
Las Vegas Night with Her Best Friend

Visit the Author Profile page
at Harlequin.com for more titles.

To my family, as always. I love you!

PROLOGUE

SAMUEL GRANT SWALLOWED as the heavy metallic clang of a door sliding shut came from somewhere beyond his line of sight. He knew what was coming, if not now, then soon enough. Skipping school to attend that protest march had probably not been the smartest move, but his closest friends had done the same thing. Then fists started flying and the same friends who'd urged him to come with them ditched him the second the police pulled up in their cruisers.

Sam blew out a breath. He would have fled too, if not for the elderly man who'd fallen after being jostled by the crowd. Sam had reached down to help him up and waited with him until he was steady on his feet, a photo he'd dropped now clutched in his weathered hand. As soon as the man started walking away, though, Sam had felt a hand on his arm. He knew instinctively that it wasn't to help him but to restrain him from leaving.

Voices traveled down the gray hallway, reaching him. The one he recognized made him close his eyes for a moment. It looked like the inevitable was going to happen right now.

He braced himself, tilting his chin in a belligerent move that belied the pounding of his heart. Then his dad appeared on the other side of the bars.

Carter Grant stared at him for a long time without saying a word, and for an instant he wondered if his dad was just going to leave him in there. His way of teaching his rebellious son a lesson, maybe. Just like so many other lessons he'd had over the years. People who said money could buy happiness were wrong. So very wrong.

Because Sam wasn't happy. And from looking at his dad's face, those steely eyes and tight set of his jaw which contained a mixture of anger and exasperation, he doubted his father was happy either.

Maybe that was partly Sam's doing. But certainly not all of it.

"Go ahead and open the door." His dad's voice was steady…the low tones gave nothing away. Not a good sign.

The guard murmured something into the device he held in his hand. A second later, the door slid open with a grinding of gears that made his teeth hurt. Sam was pretty sure he was going to hear that sound in his dreams. It was also a wake-up call. There had to be a better way to assert his ideas than constantly going head-to-head with his father. But he had no idea what that might be. Or how to go about it.

His dad motioned him out but said nothing as they walked down the hallway. He said nothing as the officer at a desk handed Sam his cell phone and wallet and a few other belongings. And he said nothing on the long ride home. But as their driver pulled up in front of the huge, exorbitant home Sam had grown up in in Manhattan, his dad held up a finger, telling him to wait.

And so he did, although the urge to burst from the car and sprint to his room was strong. But no. He was going to face the music this time.

The man who'd raised him turned to face him. "Anything to say for yourself?"

Sam had a lot to say, actually, but nothing that would do him any good, nor did he want it to, so he just shrugged.

His dad pinched the bridge of his nose between his thumb and fingers and sighed. "So be it. But you're not to come out of your room for the next week, except to go to school and come home. And I will check with the school to make sure you are where you're supposed to be."

A week was nothing. Sam was surprised his punishment wasn't longer, seeing as he'd been arrested, but because he was only fifteen, he'd been sent to juvenile hall rather than placed in a holding cell with adults. "I will be."

The truth was Sam didn't want to wind up in jail. He could help no one from there. So he'd better figure out another way to go about things before he did something that might cost him more than a mere week of restriction.

"See that you are." His dad sighed before adding, "And I'd rather you don't tell your brother and sister and especially not your mother what kind of trouble you've gone and gotten yourself into this time. You make straight A's, for God's sake. So why do you always feel the need to buck my authority?"

It wasn't like Sam had ever done anything like this before. He didn't "buck authority." At least not his teachers or coaches. If he was honest, it was just his dad. And it was usually just stuff that he knew would irritate the hell out of him.

Sam had no idea why he did it, so all he could do was just give his father another shrug.

"Are you at least going to keep quiet about it to your mom?"

"I won't say anything to anyone." Not to his mom, sister or his older brother or his teachers. But what he was going to do was find another way to make a difference in this world. Something that wouldn't get him sent to juvie or get him into hot water like it had today. Or at least he hoped that it wouldn't.

"Good. Now, let's get you inside. I'm sure Theresa has set something aside for your dinner." The family's housekeeper had been a godsend for Sam and was used to his parents' absence, since they had obligations almost every single day. Running a mega corporation and being the head of a large charitable organization took a lot of time and energy. Energy that left the Grant kids with a lot of time on their hands.

Sam got out of the car, aware that his father had also exited and was following close behind. He had expected more berating and accusations than what had happened. But that didn't mean that this was going to blow over like the rest of his stunts had. No, he was pretty sure this was going to come back and bite him in the butt when he least expected it to.

But he deserved it. He'd done what he'd done and couldn't expect there to be no consequences. So for the next week, he was going to do what he could to stay out of trouble. But one thing was for sure—in three years, when he turned eighteen, he was getting out. Out of the house, out of Manhattan and maybe even out of the United States.

He didn't know what that would look like yet, but anything was better than being the richest kid at a school filled with other rich kids. Soon he would be out from under that cloud and on his own. Then he could start helping people who couldn't help themselves. How he would do that without money was yet to be seen. But he'd find a way.

Or at least he hoped that he would.

CHAPTER ONE

LUCINDA GALEANO ENTERED the small conference room, her nerves on edge. She and a handful of other people at the hospital were being given the opportunity to join a groundbreaking team that combined microsurgery, physical therapy, plastic surgery and a few other specialties that would help people with facial paralysis. It was funded by a grant from some big corporation that she'd never heard of and would be called the Manhattan Memorial Hospital Pediatric Microsurgery and Facial-Reanimation Department. They had brought in some outside doctor to head up the project, and everyone would be meeting him. He'd evidently been at the hospital for a few weeks already, but since she'd only recently been asked to join the team, she had no idea who he was. Lucy thought she'd read the name somewhere—in a flyer, maybe it had been mentioned when she'd been called in to talk with the hospital administrator—but hell if she could remember it now. The name hadn't mattered. The opportunity had. And it had come at the perfect time.

Her gaze swept the room before frowning. Except for a man with his back to her who seemed to be perusing some sort of pamphlet, she was the first one there. She glanced at her watch… hmmm…there were still twenty minutes until the meeting actually started. Lucy's foot collided with something—a chair?—and a mad scramble to maintain her grip on the coffee in her hand ensued. The coffee won as the cup flew a few feet and landed on the table in front of her, the lid popping off and sloshing scalding liquid everywhere, including the front of her new scrubs, the ones with bright blue parrots all over them.

Before she could stop herself, she swore long and loud, the stream of words in her mother tongue spewing through the room in a fury every bit as hot as her coffee. She stared at the mess she'd made. It had already been a chaotic day, and to add this…

At least no one had been sitting at that table. She glanced around to see if there were any paper towels at the nearby refreshment table.

"Dejame ayudarte con eso."

The soft words murmured in accented Spanish made her head jerk to the side. The man who'd been at the front of the room now stood next to her, a handful of the paper towels she'd been looking for gripped in his strong hand. And his eyes… She swallowed. They were bluer than anything she could remember seeing and held an amusement that should have made her anger go up another notch. But instead it defused all of her irritation, and she shut her own eyes, mentally switching her language to English. Then she peered up at him, nose crinkling as she finally saw the humor in the situation.

"Tell me you didn't understand a thing I said a second ago."

"Every single word of it, and let me tell you… I'm shocked."

Except he wasn't, and that made her laugh. And that surprised her as much as his words had. "I'm sorry. Not everyone understands Spanish, so it's been a habit to confine my more—er, colorful language—to something other than English."

"Colorful language. It definitely contained a few hues I recognized. And some that are new to me." A smile cracked the right side of his face, fascinating her and sending a flare of heat through her midsection. What would it look like if he fully embraced that smile? She bit her lip. Better not to even think about that.

She smirked. "I guess I should sort out those colors before letting them leave my mouth."

The heat in her belly grew, and she studied him under her lashes, liking everything that she saw. What was wrong with her?

Remember the last time you let a stranger affect you that way?

It ended with a note left on her pillow a month before her wedding day.

So she counted from one to twenty. In Spanish. Non-colorful Spanish.

One of his brows went up. "Great strategy. I'll have to remember that."

For a split second, she thought she'd counted out loud rather than in her head, then realized he was talking about what she'd said about her cursing. *¡Dios!* She was going to have to watch herself around this one. She wondered which department he worked in.

She tried to take the paper towels from him to clean up the coffee, but he did it for her, sweeping up the liquid with a speed that was impressive. As was just about everything about the man, from the straight sandy hair that fell over his forehead to the tanned forearms revealed by the rolled sleeves of his blue button-down shirt. Lord have mercy, she was treading on dangerous ground here.

But at least it had jolted her from any painful memories. At least for the moment. So she could forgive herself for noticing something... anything...that didn't have to do with her fiancé's sudden change of heart. *Ex*-fiancé.

He finished cleaning up and then threw the towels into a nearby trash can before coming back over to her, right hand outstretched. "Sam Grant, and you are?"

The name rang a bell, and right now that bell was clanging an alarm that she couldn't ignore. But neither could she avoid shaking the man's hand, so she put her fingers in his and introduced herself. "I'm Lucy Galeano."

Wait. There was a Logan Grant here at the hospital who was the head of the neonatal surgical unit. He'd just gotten back together with his ex-wife, from what she'd heard. Could they be related? Not likely. Grant was a fairly common surname here in the States. Kind of like Suarez in Paraguay, where her parents were from. And if Logan's brother was working here at the hospital, surely she would have heard about it. Or their paths would have crossed.

"Ah, you must be our pediatric physical therapist. Welcome."

The authority with which he said that made her release his hand in a hurry and take a step back. But now there were other people filing into the room and taking seats. With a nod, he went back to the front of the room where MMH's administrator joined him, shaking Sam's hand. But she'd bet Todd Wells's palm wouldn't tingle the way hers was still doing.

She rolled the name around in her head over and over, trying to figure it out as she took one of the few seats that were now left. It looked like there were fifteen people who would be on the team.

Todd went to where the U-shaped configuration of tables opened up. He welcomed them to the exciting new team that was one of only a few medical centers embarking in this new field. "And it was the only way we could lure one of our medical school alumni, back from Uruguay, where he's just opened a clinic specializing in some of the things we hope to do. Everyone, please welcome the head of our team, Sam Grant," Todd said. "He arrived a few weeks ago, so some of you may have met him at our fundraising gala. Most of you know of his family, who funded a wing of this hospital. And of course, he is the brother of our own Logan Grant over in the neonatal department."

Dios Santo. He *was* related to Logan. And Sam was the new head of the team? Her mind zeroed in on the name, and yes, now she remembered it had been on that flyer. In bold print.

What on earth would he think of her? All that stuff about swearing in Spanish and sloshing her coffee all over the table? Was he wondering how on earth he could trust her with children who required precise, delicate care?

She hoped not. This was her dream job. She loved working with kids but longed to do something beyond physical therapy for broken wrists or sprained ankles. And to work with complex facial muscles was the chance of a lifetime. Would he now have her thrown off the team and replaced?

As soon as this was over, Lucy was going to go up to him and apologize. One for not recognizing his name. And two for letting her temper get the best of her. She never ever lost her cool with her young patients. But from now on, every interaction she had with this man was going to be schooled. Every smile, every frown, every word was going to be analyzed before she let it happen.

At least she hoped it would. In reality, if she couldn't keep her emotions in check, then maybe she didn't deserve to be on this team.

The hell she didn't! And to even let herself think along those lines was to invite disaster.

One she was going to do everything in her power to avoid. Because she did deserve to be here. She'd worked her butt off to prove to herself and everyone else that she was good at her job. And to be invited to join this group of top professionals was something she'd only dreamed of. So she was going to prove to Sam Grant and everyone else that they'd picked the exact right person for this exact right job. No matter what it took.

Sam tensed the second Todd Wells mentioned his family and the grant his father had given to the hospital. He'd been so careful to make sure the offer from Manhattan Memorial hadn't been orchestrated by his father. He'd even called Logan to ask his advice and see if he'd heard anything. He hadn't, and Carter Grant hadn't said anything to him about trying to get Sam back to New York.

And Todd Wells had confirmed that they'd gotten his name from a colleague who'd heard of his work at the clinic in Uruguay.

Fortunately their sister was poised to take up the reins of the corporation, since neither Sam nor Logan were interested in running their father's business. And Sam actually hadn't heard from his dad once in the two years he'd been in Uruguay, other than in the perfunctory birthday text messages his mom sent him. They'd always said that his father sent his love. He didn't believe it—after all his dad had never used those words with him and probably never would.

He knew at some point he'd run into at least his mom here at the hospital since one of her charity works had her doing a weekly story reading to the children in the oncology department. And he'd asked Logan not to say anything to them until he at least got situated. But then Todd had asked him to go to the fundraiser which had happened not long after he'd arrived back in the States, and of course his mom and dad had been there. He'd been forced to say hello, but his parents had been called to greet someone else almost immediately, and that had been that.

He shook his family from his thoughts as he tried to remember why he was here. It was far too soon to be having second thoughts about leaving Uruguay. Even though it had come at the perfect time. He'd broken up with Priscilla, the woman he'd lived with for the last five years.

She'd been the reason he'd gone to Uruguay in the first place, since her family was all there. But then he'd overheard a quiet conversation between her and her mother about the money he'd inherited from his grandfather, and something in his gut had curdled. And when he decided to donate it all to start a clinic specializing in children who needed facial surgery, she'd balked and tried to talk him out of it. And even though she now worked at that very same clinic, it had been the beginning of the end. There'd been many arguments before he finally moved out of their shared apartment and got on a plane heading back to the States a year and a half after the clinic opened.

But to return to Manhattan? It hadn't even been on his radar, until that offer had come in.

His eyes landed on Lucy Galeano. Lucy had to be short for something. At least he thought it might be. Lucinda? Luciana? And although she spoke Spanish, her accent was different from what he'd heard in Uruguay.

It didn't matter where she was from. She was on his team—thanks to him—and he'd be working with her. The less curious he was about her as a person, the better it would be for both of them.

He'd already tried having a romance with someone he worked with…someone he'd lived and breathed hospital life with. In the end, it hadn't worked out—and probably wouldn't have even if he hadn't overheard that conversation. Because although he'd cared for Priscilla, he'd discovered his parents' influence on him as a child had been more powerful than he'd imagined. He had a hard time investing himself emotionally because he'd never experienced much of that. Except with people like coaches and teachers. Priscilla had seemed to give it her all, but even she hadn't been able to make up for his deficit. In the end, his family's money had tainted what he'd believed about their relationship. And it cemented the idea that keeping his distance emotionally—even when it came to romantic partners—was the right thing to do. At least for him. That way no one got hurt.

He'd do well to remember that.

Sam didn't remember much about what he said in his speech to the group, but thankfully he'd had notes to rely on as he explained what he hoped to accomplish as a team. He was glad he'd opted to keep things short and to the point and was happy to hand the meeting back over to Todd, keeping his attention firmly on the man this time. The administrator was much more eloquent than Sam had been as he gave his closing remarks. Then again it was the man's job to be persuasive, just as it had been his dad's job when it came to running a company.

But Sam wasn't running an empire or even a clinic anymore. All he wanted to do was help people. He just hoped he didn't come to regret working in a place where his dad had waved his magic wand and made a hospital wing appear out of thin air. All it had taken was money. A whole lot of money.

"Are there any questions for Dr. Grant?" The administrator's question made him tense all over again. He hadn't really expected a question-and-answer session, since he wasn't exactly sure how things were going to work at this point. He much preferred to call people into his office one at a time and discuss expectations on both sides. Sam didn't shrink from hard conversations, but he preferred that those happen in private.

And any future meetings with Lucy Galeano?

His jaw tightened. They would be exactly the same as all of his other meetings. Professional and to the point. Just like his speech. None of the people in this room had officially signed a written contract yet. That wouldn't happen until he could feel them out—he wanted to handpick his own team and had made that clear to Todd, who'd agreed. The administrator had simply offered to be a filter, bringing in people he thought would be a good fit. And Lucy's bio seemed to be perfect. But if she didn't fit the bill for what he was looking for, he needed to be objective enough to say so. And right now, he was not at all objective. Because all he could hear in his head was the sexy huskiness of her voice as she'd let those words tumble from her lips. Very pink lips with very…

Get a grip! He was just months out from his relationship with Pri, and he did not need to be thinking of anyone like that.

Surprisingly, there were no questions, and the meeting was soon dismissed. Several people came up to shake his hand and express their excitement about the hospital's newest program, but his attention was on Lucy, who was hanging out at the back of the room, looking very much like she was waiting to have a word with him but preferred not to do that in front of everyone else.

Why?

That innocent back-and-forth banter they'd had before the meeting came to mind. He hoped she hadn't taken things out of context and was hoping he'd ask her out. Maybe he needed to set the record straight. And Todd had mentioned his family's money and its contribution to the hospital. But Sam had let that portion of his life go when he'd opened the clinic. So if, like Priscilla, she had dollar signs in her eyes she'd be sorely disappointed when she found out the truth.

The last person left, and Lucy made her way up to him, picking her steps with care this time. He had no idea what he was going to say if she really did think he was attracted to her. Because, hell, he had been, and she'd probably been able to see it immediately.

"Um… Dr. Grant…about earlier…" Her words faded away, but the fact that she'd addressed him by his title made a few of his muscles relax.

"What about it?" The words came out a little more curt than he'd meant them to, but then he felt out of his element right now.

"I hope it won't affect the way you see me as a physical therapist. I don't normally go around cussing."

It wasn't what he'd expected her to say, and he couldn't stop his smile, a sense of relief washing over him. So this was what she was worried about?

"At least not in English." He went on, "It's fine. I've read about your work with children and have to say I was very impressed. I asked that you be added to the team. Although we won't make that official until I meet with you one-on-one."

"You asked for me? I wondered why I'd been added to the roster just two weeks ago."

He had, but he normally wasn't great with names. The fact that he'd known who she was the second she'd introduced herself was strange. If it were anyone else who'd been in the room, would he have? Probably not just from reading their bio.

"We'll need someone whose patience can be tested and who isn't easily rattled. At least unless there's coffee involved." His smile switched back on, which wasn't like him. But there was something about this woman that made him want to tease her into some kind of reaction.

The type of reaction he was after was the only thing in question.

"Hot coffee is my weakness. I needed that shot of caffeine, you know."

"Afraid I'd put you to sleep?"

Her teeth came down on her lip before she said, "That wasn't what I meant. I actually needed something to distract me from…"

She'd been about to add something before stopping. He'd never know what unless he asked her, and he wasn't about to do that.

He decided to put her mind at ease. "Don't worry about it. Things are fine, if that's what you're worried about."

"I kind of was. I thought maybe an apology was in order."

"Not at all. I think it was just what I needed— the reminder that we all are human, that we all have our weaknesses."

Her brows went up. "Even you?"

"Especially me." The longer he was around her, the more he realized that just because he'd ended one relationship, it didn't mean he was immune to all women. He wasn't. Lucy was proving that to be true, and he wasn't sure why. It was time to cut this conversation short until he could figure that out. "So if there's nothing else…?"

She blinked once, twice before her brows came together. "Um…no. Nothing else. I assume you'll let us know exactly what you need?"

He didn't want to look too closely at those words.

"Yep, I'll be getting together with everyone soon and hashing out roles and making formal offers."

"Within our particular specialties, right?"

"Can you think of another way to do it?"

She shook her head. "No. Not at this moment, but if I do, I'll let you know."

Damn. He realized he was smiling again. Lucy was too much for him to deal with right now. Maybe in a few days after he'd talked to some other people on the team, his head would be clearer. The only thing he was sure of was that the longer he stood there, the more he'd be smiling, and that was not what he wanted to do. With anyone.

"You do that. I'll set up a meeting with you in a few days, if that's okay, and get your thoughts on the new department." In case she got the wrong idea, he quickly added, "I plan on doing the same thing with all the folks who were here today."

"Understood. Let me know if you need me to do anything before then."

That was another sentence he wasn't going to touch with a ten-foot pole. So with one last smile—one of the fake smiles that he hated so much—he bid her farewell. "I'm sure I'll see you around."

How stupid was that as a get-me-out-of-here tactic? But it was evidently effective, since she gave a nod of her head and spun on her heel leaving the room. It was then that he realized the printing all over her scrubs had been parrots with tiny conversation bubbles over their heads that read *Repeat after me* inscribed in black ink. Prophetic, no? Because he was about to find himself saying that over and over in his dealings with her.

Which he did, the moment she left the room. "Repeat after me—no more getting involved with anyone from work." He was going to be saying that a lot over the next couple of days, until it was emblazoned on his brain in as many languages as he could muster. Until he actually believed it was true.

CHAPTER TWO

IT HAD BEEN three days since the team introductions, and Lucy hadn't heard from Sam yet, but then again he'd said he would be meeting with them over the next few days, so it hadn't been that long. She couldn't help wondering where she fell on that list and whether or not it was significant that she hadn't been one of the first names he'd picked out of his proverbial hat. Or that she'd been notified of her place on the team much later than most of the other folks. But he said he'd asked for her specifically, so there was that.

Being notified at the last minute seemed to be a normal part of her life. Like not having any idea her fiancé was having second thoughts about marrying her until almost the last minute. Did she matter so little to people? Or was it that her cheerful manner made them think that she could handle anything and everything? Because she couldn't. And his actions had made her insecure about who she was. She now found herself having to give herself pep talks more frequently than she should have.

Like she was doing right now?

Her next patient was a five-year-old child who had fallen in kindergarten a few days ago and had complained of pain in his right hand and forearm. X-rays had shown no fractures, and so the consensus was that he had a soft-tissue injury. The recommendation was physical therapy since the pain was ongoing. It was hard in a patient this young because the tendency was to protect the injured area to avoid pain, and so at times those little guys could make the problem worse and affect their range of motion. And the mom said it was affecting his fine motor skills.

While the boy's mom watched from a nearby chair, Devon hunched in front of Lucy, a blank coloring book on the table in front of him. Although he wasn't engaging in the activity in a physical way, he was very interested in the pictures. She decided to take a different tack.

"Okay, Devon, we're going to play some different games, okay?" She frowned at the long-sleeved shirt and glanced at the boy's mother. "Do you mind if we take his shirt off? I want to watch how his arm moves as we do some exercises."

"Anything. I just want him to feel better."

She turned her attention back to the child. "Are you okay if we do that?"

He nodded but didn't say anything.

"Can you show me where it hurts, so I can be careful with it?"

Devon moved his left hand over an area that encompassed his wrist and about halfway up his forearm. "Here."

The wrist explained why he was hesitant to color, since his mom said he normally loved art and coloring. They were doing scissor work in school, and the teacher relayed that Devon cried every time he had to cut something, which was another reason he was here.

"All right. Can you lift your arms straight over your head so I can slide your shirt up?" She demonstrated the movement for him, and Devon copied it without a hitch. Another reason why she'd wanted to take the shirt off. So, there was no shoulder involvement that she could see.

She eased the shirt over his head, taking care with his injured wrist and hand. "There, that should make it easier for you." Lucy smiled at him as she folded his shirt and handed it to his mom. "Okay, let's start our games."

She pulled two sock puppets out of a drawer. One was a dog with long droopy ears and brown-

and-white spots; the other was a duck, complete with beak and soft feathers. "Which one would you like?"

The boy smiled for the first time since he arrived. "The dog. He's funny."

"He is. Do you want to name him?"

Devon tilted his head. "Spot." He pointed at the puppet using his left hand. "Because he has spots."

"Good choice."

It was telling that he was using his nondominant hand. Getting him to do anything with his right hand might be tricky. She picked up her puppet. "I think I'll call my duck Quack."

"That's silly."

"It is, because Quack is a silly guy. Now, we'll use the puppets in a minute, but I want you to do some things with this hand." She put her fingers on the boy's wrist, using a bit of pressure and watching closely. He didn't flinch. So the pain must've come from movement rather than pressure.

"I—I don't want to." His voice quivered a bit, showing his anxiety.

"I know. It hurts, doesn't it?"

He nodded.

"But I want to try to help it feel better. Will you let me help you?" Lucy pulled out a chart of faces, represented by yellow circles. The circles ranged from a large smile and traveled to a face that was crying. "You can tell me how much each activity hurts, okay?"

She'd normally be able to tell through his reactions, but some children were more stoic than others. Plus Lucy wanted Devon to be able to express his own pain level regardless of how much she could tell as they went through the exercises.

He nodded. "But you won't hurt it."

"I won't touch your hand unless I tell you I'm going to, okay?" She smiled again to reassure him.

"Okay."

"I want you to copy what I do. First I want you to hold out both hands in front of you, then we're going to close our hands like this." She made both of her hands into loose fists. "Can you do this?"

Devon did the left one effortlessly, but he was slower with the right one. But he was able to curl his fingers and get them to close.

She then had him point to the chart to say how much that had hurt. Not too much, judging from the face he chose. It was a closed-mouth smile.

"Very good. Now we're both going to put our hands on the table like this." She put her hands flat on the table, fingers splayed apart. Devon copied her. "Okay, this might be a little harder, but try to do what I do. Let's lift our pinkies."

Lucy raised both little fingers, keeping the rest of her digits where they were.

Devon had no problem doing this, raising his fingers. He did the same with the rest of them as she slowly worked her way to where she suspected the pain was. When she lifted her index fingers Devon only did it with his left hand.

"Can you do it with your other hand too?"

"It'll hurt." That quavery in his voice returned.

"How much do you think it will hurt?"

He pointed to the crying face on the chart, again using his left hand.

"That bad, huh?"

He nodded.

She thought for a minute. If his index finger hurt to lift, it stood to reason that the ligament that controlled the movement was inflamed, since it traveled part way up the forearm. "Can I touch your finger?"

Devon shook his head to say no.

"How about Quack. Can he touch it?" She slid the puppet onto her hand, glancing up as a movement at the door caught her eye. Her heart seized for a minute before starting up again. Sam Grant was standing just inside the physical therapy room, his gaze catching and holding hers as he leaned against the wall and crossed his arms over his chest. Was he checking up on her? Well, she wasn't going to let him rattle her. She was going to do her job the same way she always did it.

"Maybe. He won't hurt it, will he?"

"No, he won't hurt it." If what she suspected was true, his finger wouldn't hurt if someone else made it go up, it would only hurt if Devon tried to initiate the movement himself. If that was the case, some anti-inflammatories and icing it could take down the swelling and help it heal.

"Okay, Quack, you heard Devon. You can touch his finger, but be very, very careful." She was hyperaware of Sam not twenty yards away. And although the room tended to be noisy with an array of different patients and therapists, she had no doubt that he could hear every word she said.

Lucy had the puppet touch the boy's finger, running his beak up the digit and following the path she knew the ligament traveled. "Is this where it hurts?"

"It doesn't hurt now."

"I know. But is this where it would hurt if you lifted your finger?"

He nodded.

This was a boy of few words. But that was okay. He was actually doing great. Some children really disliked the process, which was how she'd discovered that the puppets could often do what she as a person couldn't.

She took the puppet off. "Do you think Spot could keep Quack company for a minute while I get something?"

Lucy was tempted to go over to see what Sam wanted, but her patient came first. She helped the boy put the duck puppet on, not batting an eye when he took his own puppet off first rather than letting her put it on his right hand. That was okay. She just wanted to get a ruler to see if he would let Quack lift that finger using a flat object.

She went over to where the equipment was kept and grabbed a small plastic school-type ruler. She'd chosen yellow to match her puppet. As she was walking back to the table where Devon sat with his back to her, she could hear Spot "talking" to Quack. Then she frowned as something caught her eye. What was that on his lower back? A mark of some kind.

She got closer and squatted down to get a better look. Devon's skin was mottled with red over his lumbar spine. Midline, actually. "I'm right behind you, Devon. Does your back hurt at all?"

"No."

She slid on an exam glove from a nearby drawer and touched the area, using gentle pressure to assess it. It was completely flat, looking almost rash-like but having no raised edges. She glanced at his mom. "Has he always had this red patch on his back?"

"Yes. We always just thought it was a birthmark. Why?"

"No particular reason." Staying where she was, she went on, "How did Devon hurt his hand—do you know?"

"They said he was running and his feet seemed to get tangled together, and he fell." His mother shook her head. "He actually falls quite a bit when he's not paying attention to what he's doing."

A chill went over her. "Devon, do your legs or feet ever hurt?"

He shrugged.

It wasn't a no. But it also wasn't a yes. She bit her lip, hesitating.

Her glance went back to his mother. "How often would you say he falls?"

"I don't know exactly. Every couple of days. He's an active kid. Is it important?"

"Not necessarily." She stood and caught Sam's eye and motioned him over. She knew he was a plastic surgeon and not a neurologist, but she could use another set of eyes right now. Hopefully he would tell her she was overreacting. But she'd had some very personal experience with childhood spinal issues. Her older sister, Bella, had been born with a neural tube defect that had needed to be corrected. It was why they'd come to the States from Paraguay.

And Lucy had been deeply involved in helping her sister work on her PT exercises even as a child, idolizing the people who came to the house to help with therapy. It was one of the reasons she'd become a physical therapist herself.

So yes, she was probably seeing things that weren't there. But if she wasn't… And if Devon fell or moved just the wrong way and her gut feeling was right, it could have devastating consequences.

Sam came over immediately. When she knelt back down beside Devon, he followed suit. "What do you make of this?"

Devon's mom stood and came over to look at what they were doing. "Is something wrong?"

Thankfully the boy was still playing with the puppets and wasn't paying much attention to what they were doing.

She forced herself to smile at Devon's mom.

"This is Dr. Grant. I just wanted him to look at this mark. You said he's had it since birth?"

"Well, I always thought so. I didn't actually notice it until he was a month old. He was a preemie and stayed in the hospital for three weeks. I pointed it out to his pediatrician—in Arkansas, where we moved from—and he thought it was just a birthmark too, since all of Devon's scores were within normal ranges."

"I'm only pointing it out now because of where the mark is located and the mention of frequent falls. It might be nothing."

Sam glanced at her and nodded as if saying he understood what she was thinking. He stood and turned toward Devon's mom. "Would you mind if I have one of my colleagues come down and take a look, if he's available? Your son has never had an MRI of his spine?"

"His spine? No. He's never complained of back pain to me. But if you think that mark might mean something, then yes, please let anyone you want look at it."

"Thanks," he said. "I'll be back in just a moment."

Lucy put her hand on the mom's shoulder and gave a gentle squeeze. "Let's not worry until there's something to worry about."

"Okay." But the woman didn't look convinced.

She couldn't blame her. If Devon were her child, she'd be plenty worried. Lucy was concerned, and the boy wasn't even hers.

"Let's get back to the session." Lucy sat down with Devon. "See this little ruler I have here?"

"Yes."

"If I can have Quack back, I'm going to have him slide it under this finger." She touched his index finger. "He won't do anything with it unless I tell him to. And I'll tell you and Spot first."

"Will it hurt?"

"I don't think so, but if it does you can tell me to stop, okay?"

"Okay."

She helped Devon put Spot back on his hand, then she donned the duck puppet.

Then she put the ruler between the duck's beak as if he were holding it. "Devon, I don't want you to move your hand or fingers while Quack does this. Just let them rest."

"Can I keep Spot with me?"

"Yes, of course. He can help you. And he can help Quack." She had the puppet carefully slide the ruler beneath the boy's index finger, turning it so that only that particular digit was lying on the thin plastic. She leaned down as if whispering something to Quack and nodding as if the puppet had answered her. "Quack wants to lift the ruler just a little. Your finger will go up too. Are you ready?"

His face became anxious again. "It's gonna hurt!"

"I don't think it will," she said again. "But if it does we'll stop."

His mom slid closer and put her arm around his thin shoulders. "You can do this, Dev. I'm right here with you."

He didn't say anything else, so using the puppet, Lucy lifted his finger about a centimeter off the table. "Does that hurt?"

Devon shook his head. "Good." When Lucy lifted it a little higher, repeating the question, Devon again indicated it didn't hurt.

"Very good." She lowered the ruler and slid it out from under the boy's hand.

She did a few more exercises with Devon and found that his wrist didn't hurt unless his index finger was in use. It looked to be a much simpler injury than the report or her exam indicated. She would check with his pediatrician, but she would bet that he jammed the finger when he fell and the ligament used when the digit was raised was inflamed. It could be almost as painful as a fracture. Especially to a child who didn't understand why something in his body hurt.

"I think it's just in his index finger. I'm going

to call his pediatrician and ask about taking an anti-inflammatory and using ice on the area."

His mom hugged him and then looked at her. "That's great news. But what about his back?"

Lucy glanced up to see that Sam was heading their way. When he arrived, he said, "Dr. Asbury is with a patient and can't come down at the moment, but we can put you in an exam room and he'll take a look as soon as he has a minute. Are you in a rush to get anywhere?"

"He would normally be going to his T-ball practice, but since his hand still hurts a lot, we decided to skip it today. So we have time."

T-ball. Lucy tried to contain her shudder. One of those games that could very well cause a lot of damage if that mark indicated what she thought it might.

"I think that's a good call," Sam said. "I'll take you up there."

He glanced at Lucy, who shook her head, although there was nowhere she'd rather be right now than in that room with her patient. "I have another appointment in fifteen minutes." She smiled at Devon and thought for a minute. "But hopefully I'll see you next week. Do you want to take Spot with you until then?"

"Could I?" The boy's words were filled with

excitement, and he held the puppet close to his chest as if cradling a real puppy.

"Of course you can." She turned to her own puppet. "Tell them bye, Quack."

"Quack. Quack." Lucy made the noises as duck-like as she could muster.

When she glanced at Sam, she saw he was trying not to smile. So she added another *"Quack!"* for good measure.

This time the man did smile. "You did that on purpose," he murmured for her ears only.

"*I* didn't do it. Quack did."

Sam rolled his eyes. "I'd like to talk to you a little bit later. Let me know when you have an opening in your schedule."

"Okay."

The trio left the therapy area, and all of her anxieties rose to the surface again. An opening in her schedule? Was that why he'd come down here? Was he having second thoughts about her being on the team?

Surely not. That wouldn't make any sense. But she didn't have time to worry about it right now. She had another patient to get ready for.

Lucy cleared her desk and sanitized the space Devon had occupied before opening the big drawer at the bottom of her desk where she kept about ten puppets. They almost always put her more nervous patients at ease. And she did a lot of role-play with them on injuries, having the child sometimes act out how he or she had been hurt. She started to stuff Quack in there with the rest of them but paused, giving the puppet a stern look. "If you hurt my chances for being on that team, you and I are going to have a long talk."

The puppet didn't make a sound. But Lucy could have sworn the thing looked at her with a sly grin before she dropped him into the drawer and quickly slammed it shut.

Greg Asbury saw them almost immediately. Sam had stayed because he was curious about what the mark might mean. He'd already deduced what Lucy thought it could indicate: tethered cord syndrome.

Tethered cord syndrome was a close relative of spina bifida—also known as neural tube defect—but rather than having a portion of the spinal cord that hadn't closed during gestation, a tethered cord occurred when part of the spinal cord attached to another structure, in this case the skin of the lower back. It was a fairly rare finding. But the discoloration was one of a cluster of symptoms that could occur with the syndrome, like an anomaly of the skin, whether a dimpling or a hemangioma. There were even cases where patches of hair grew in the spot where the cord was tethered. Falling or leg weakness or pain were also symptoms. Some people lived with a tethered cord their whole lives without knowing it. But if it were taut, a quick move or injury could cause the cord to stretch past its capacity, sometimes causing irreparable damage to the nerves. Then leg weakness could become paralysis.

There was only one way to know for sure. An MRI.

Dr. Asbury did a careful examination after hearing from both Sam and Devon's mom. When he looked at the boy's back, he frowned and asked some more pointed questions about muscle weakness.

"I don't know, really. He does fall—like kids do—but other than that and sometimes having trouble keeping up with his classmates when he's running the bases in T-ball, I haven't really noticed anything. And his teachers haven't mentioned anything either."

The pediatric neurologist, who was also on Sam's team, talked about the possibility of the cord being stuck in the area where the birthmark was and asking if he could try and get Devon cleared for an MRI in the next week or so. "He can't play sports until we know for sure, so if he's involved in any..."

"Just T-ball, but I can explain to the coaches that he can't play until the test is done. If it is what you mentioned, can it be fixed?"

"Depending on how much of the cord is tethered, we can normally go in and free that portion of the tissue."

"You mean surgery."

"Yes. But it's not as involved as some of the other surgeries involving the spinal cord. We just want to make sure the vertebrae are all there and shaped the way they should be. We'll know more after the MRI."

"I take it we can't just leave it alone."

Greg took a seat next to Devon's mom, who'd introduced herself as Rachel. "I wouldn't recommend it. If he gets struck in the back by, say, a baseball or if he slides into home, for example, it could jerk the cord and not only cause a lot of pain but actually damage the cord itself. That is something we don't want happening under any circumstances."

"I see. So the sooner we have the MRI, the better. Will someone Devon's age even hold still for it to be done? He's not the most cooperative child in the world. You can ask Lucy, his physical therapist."

The mention of her name made Sam's jaw tense before he forced it to relax as Greg answered the question.

"We can sometimes give them a light sedative, if there's a lot of anxiety. We can also put children's music onto a set of headphones and let him listen to that and put a sleep mask on him to help with any claustrophobia he might feel. There are all kinds of ways to help with anxiety."

"Okay. So until then, we just wait?" Rachel asked.

"Yes." Greg put a hand on Devon's head. "His hand injury might be a blessing in disguise. From what you said he doesn't want to use it."

"No, he doesn't."

"Well, that might work to our advantage. So try to just keep him calm. I imagine by next Monday we'll have our answer."

"Okay. Is there anything else?" she asked.

Greg smiled. "Yes. Go home and try not to worry. If it's a tethered cord, we've caught it fairly early. That's a good thing."

Her lips twisted. "I'll take your word for it. But thank you for seeing us. Devon, can you tell Dr. Grant and Dr. Asbury goodbye?"

The boy held up his puppet, and like Lucy had done, he had it bark a goodbye.

Once they were out of the room, Greg clapped

Sam on the shoulder. "That was a good catch. Not everyone would have seen that mark or realized what it could mean."

"It actually wasn't me. It was the physical therapist who'll be on our pediatric microsurgery team."

"Ah… Lucy Galeano. She is extremely good at her job. They send all of the tough PT cases her way."

Something about the way the man said that made Sam look a little bit closer, but he saw nothing but sincerity in the neurosurgeon's face. Besides, there was a ring on the other doctor's left hand.

And if there was something more there? It was none of his business as long as it didn't affect either's professionalism while on the job. He didn't want any kind of messy publicity damaging the new program before it even got off the ground.

Since when did he worry about things like that? He thought his parents' hypersensitivity about the media would have burned that out of him long ago. Maybe there was a little bit of them in him after all. Logan seemed to have made his peace with their father, and their sister had embraced the company and all it stood for. But as long as Carter Grant stayed out of Sam's way and didn't try to interfere with his work at the hospital, they would stick with whatever uneasy truce they'd had over these last several years. They weren't friends, nor were they ever likely to be. But he could deal with the way things were.

At least for now.

CHAPTER THREE

LUCY TRIED TO rein in her curiosity, but it finally got the better of her. She hadn't heard from Sam about Devon, and she really didn't want to wait another day to hear if they'd found something or not. Or maybe they hadn't even scheduled an MRI. Maybe the neurologist had brushed off her fears as unfounded.

But still. A simple phone call or text to update her would have been nice.

Except she didn't think she had Sam's personal cell phone number, and he probably didn't have hers either. And did she really want to go through the hospital directory or a personal assistant, if the man even had one? Not really. Especially if it turned out her fears were unfounded. It might be reason enough for him to wonder about her qualifications for the new position.

And he'd never told her exactly why he'd come down to the PT department in the first place.

It was driving her crazy, and she could only think of one way to quiet her thoughts.

Lucy could venture up to the fourth floor and see if he was in his office. She could always use the pretext of wanting to give him that date he'd asked for.

Well, not a date as in going out to dinner, but he'd asked her for some openings in her schedule. Which she now had after looking at it for what seemed like hours and then screwing up the courage to actually enter some dates and times into her phone.

She wasn't sure about seeing him face-to-face, although if she was going to work with the man, she was going to have to get over her reservations. The smile he'd given her after she'd made those silly duck sounds had thrown her for a loop. She'd wanted to see a full smile ever since he'd cranked up that one side of his mouth during the initial team meeting. Well, she'd finally gotten that smile, and the combination of white teeth and tiny lines beside his eyes had made her mouth go dry. She couldn't have quacked again if her life depended on it.

She left her puppet in the drawer this time and went to the elevator, taking a deep breath and forcing herself to push the button to go up. She'd never actually had a need to go to the plastic sur-

gery department. And although she'd heard that
Sam didn't deal with adult surgeries and only
specialized in pediatric corrective procedures,
she still wondered if he would dissect someone's
looks and find them lacking in areas. How many
before-and-after pictures had he seen during his
training? And how many insecurities had driven
people to seek out surgery?

Lucy had her own insecurities. Especially
now.

That was ridiculous. People chose to straighten
or whiten their teeth all the time. Or tattooed
and pierced their bodies. And she never thought
anything of it. Her own ears were pierced, and
she had a tiny bunny tattoo on her left shoulder representing her sister, Bella. Why should
anyone be given grief for getting tummy tucks
or other elective surgeries? Just because Sam
looked pretty perfect in every way didn't mean
he judged other people on how they looked.

Like she was judging him?

Yes. She was being a hypocrite for even thinking along those lines.

Ugh. Once she arrived at the fourth floor, she
found that those thoughts melted away the moment she spotted Sam in the large waiting room
to the left. He was cradling a baby in his arms
while he talked to a woman who was probably

the mother. Even from here, she could see the baby's lip had been sutured in what looked to be a repair of some sort.

He hadn't notice her yet, and an army of butterflies gathered in her stomach, their soft wings brushing her insides in a way that felt vaguely warm...inviting. Not what butterflies normally did in these circumstances. Ugh. That had better not be her ovaries sitting up and taking notice of the scene, because she was not in the market for babies or significant others. Not after what had happened with Matt. But before that? She'd always hoped they'd have a couple of children of their own. Had looked forward to it, actually.

And then she'd found that horrible note. She'd never heard from him again. He'd left her to cancel all of the wedding plans and return gifts from the shower. It had been a singularly humiliating experience. Thank heavens her sister had been there to help her.

But the worst thing of all were the whys that kept swirling around in her head. Even now. Had he found someone else? Found something in her that was lacking...or too irritating to stand? So many questions remained unanswered. He'd never been the type of person who'd worn his heart on his sleeve, and his *I love you*s had been few and far between. But Lucy had been demonstrative enough for the both of them. Or at least she'd thought so. Maybe that had been part of the problem. But for her to have had no idea that he'd changed his mind about marrying her had been singularly crushing.

And seeing a baby just reminded her of all the hopes that had been—

Just then Sam's head turned, and he saw her. "Lucy. Hi. Are you waiting to see me?"

All she could do was nod.

She realized she was still staring when the mother's head cocked as if wondering why Lucy was just standing there. *Dios.* Every time she was around the man she seemed to make some kind of mess. Whether with her coffee or her words…or just her presence. "I can come back."

"No, just go on to my office. I'll be there shortly."

"Okay." She had no idea where the man's office even was, which was ludicrous, since that was where she'd been headed in the first place. The urge to run back to her own department came, and she had to force herself not to act on that impulse. She somehow needed to get herself under control, or she needed to just resign from the team here and now. And she didn't want to do that.

Especially after seeing that baby and knowing

that his or her life had just been changed. And Sam had played a big role in that.

This was Lucy's chance to do something big too. To help kids who might not be able to speak or smile or even chew without great difficulty. And heaven help her, she wanted to be in on that. She'd seen what could be done in Bella's case. Her sister was now a wedding planner. She was graceful and elegant, and other than her cane and a slight hitch to her gait, no one would ever know that there had been some question over whether she would ever walk. But she had. And her family owed it all to a gifted neurosurgeon who had just recently retired from his practice. Her mom still sent him a card every single year on the anniversary of Bella's surgery, thanking him for the miracle that was her daughter.

Lucy had cried on her sister's shoulder after she'd gotten that note from Matt. But Bella had walked with her through every step of undoing all the work they'd done on planning the wedding. In the end they had gone on that honeymoon cruise themselves and had laughed and drank and enjoyed life. If Matt had been that unhappy, then he'd done them both a favor by backing out. He just should have talked to her face-to-face and told her the truth rather than taking a coward's way out. But what was done was done. No matter how much she wanted to change the way it had played out, she couldn't. That was on Matt and no one else.

Lucy stopped at the nurses' desk. When one of them smiled at her and commented on her scrubs—the same ones she'd spilled coffee on a week ago—she relaxed. "Thank you. I work down in the PT department. Could you tell me where Dr. Grant's office is?"

"Which Dr. Grant? Sam or Logan? Or Harper, although she's gone by Dunn for years."

Harper? That threw her for a moment until she remembered Sam and Logan were both Grants. Maybe Harper was related to them somehow? "Sorry. *Sam* Grant."

"Got it," the woman said. "Go right down that hallway, and it'll be the third door on your left."

"Thanks."

She turned and followed the directions, finding his office right where the nurse said it would be. But she balked at going in there on her own, so she found a little waiting room a few steps away and went to sit in there. Right now it was empty. It would give her a chance to stop and collect her thoughts.

What was it about Sam that was messing with her head so much? Was it his looks? The man was undeniably gorgeous. But there were other good-looking guys at the hospital, and she'd never gotten flustered around them. Maybe the breakup was affecting how she interacted with the opposite sex more than she'd realized.

She sat and took a couple of deep, calming breaths, just like she did in yoga class. Or maybe it was that Lucy hadn't expected to see Sam holding an infant. Or to look so comfortable doing so. Even though Lucy worked with kids each and every day, none of them were babies. Even holding a friend's infant a few days ago had made her tense up, resulting in the child crying. Lucy had quickly handed the baby back. So for him to look so natural… A lump rose in her throat. He would make a great dad.

And why had that even come to mind?

Just then, the man in question rounded the corner walking right past the waiting room before backtracking and looking at her. "Why are you out here?"

She shrugged and stood. "I didn't want you to think I was ransacking your office."

Ransacking...really, Lucy?

His brow went up as he motioned her to follow him. "There's not much in there to ransack, and since I don't see a cup of coffee in your hand, there's nothing to worry about."

"Coffee?" She remembered and heat flooded her face. "Oh…*coffee.*"

He grinned and opened the door. "Come on in."

And there was that smile again. *Santa Maria*, she was in trouble.

"Sorry. I didn't realize you'd be with a patient." She sat in one of the chairs that was in front of his desk. The office was large and could be quite opulent with the right decor, but right at the moment it seemed spartan. She wasn't sure if that was surprising or not based on what she'd seen of the man. Then again, he hadn't been at the hospital that long, had he?

"Not a problem. It was just a follow-up appointment."

"I didn't realize you were already doing surgeries."

"I'm not, at least not the kinds of surgeries I hope the team will be doing. Marcus— the baby—was actually my first surgical repair at Manhattan Memorial. Now, what can I do for you? Are you here for our meeting?" He frowned. "Did we even set that up?"

"No." She felt a little more foolish for just showing up on his proverbial doorstep and decided to be honest. "I actually came to see if you'd heard anything about Devon."

"Devon?" His face cleared. "Oh, your patient from the other day. Sorry—I thought maybe Greg would have called you and let you know about the outcome. You were right. He has a tethered cord. They've already scheduled surgery to repair it. If you hadn't caught it... Well, you know what could have happened."

"I do. I have a sister who was born with spina bifida. So even though it's not the same thing, I've done quite a lot of research on spinal cord defects."

"I'm sorry. Is she okay?"

"She is, actually. She's kind and beautiful." Lucy laughed. "None of that has anything to do with her condition. Or maybe it does. She was fortunate that it could be corrected when she was still a baby. My parents made the trip to NYC after her surgeon came to Paraguay on a medical mission and arranged for them to come back to the States with him. They decided to stay in the New York area afterward. My dad was a radiologist in Paraguay and was able to get his certification to work in his field here."

"That's great. I'm glad your sister's cord defect could be corrected."

"Me too. It was a complicated surgery, but it all worked out. And I'm glad that Devon's condition can be fixed as well."

"Thanks to you."

"Thanks to Greg." She shook her head. "I just happened to notice the odd coloration. If I hadn't needed him to take his shirt off, I never would have guessed."

"He's lucky you did." Sam's eyes met hers. "I assumed you already knew the outcome of the MRI. Sorry about that. I should have checked to make sure."

"It's okay. I would have called or texted but realized I didn't know your number. Or Dr. Asbury's. And I wasn't sure about calling his office. He probably doesn't even know my name."

"Oh, he knows your name." He gave another smile, although this one didn't quite reach his eyes.

She tilted her head. "What do you mean?"

"Nothing. He just recognized that you were on our team. Greg is on it as well."

"He is? I didn't realize that. I didn't see him at the meeting." She thought for a moment. "But it makes sense that a neurosurgeon would be included. Hopefully I'll be able to really get to know the other members of the group. That initial meeting was kind of crazy and overwhelming. Actually, it was very much so."

"Yes, it was. For me as well. I still don't know a lot of people at the hospital."

Really? He'd seemed so cool and calm. "At least you know your brother. What's it like working at the same hospital as a member of your family? Is Harper your sister? One of the nurses mentioned her when I asked where Dr. Grant's office was."

"Harper is—*was*—my sister-in-law." Sam didn't say anything else for a minute, but his smile faded. "As for Logan, it's good working with him. We're close."

That was kind of a strange thing to say, especially since she didn't think she'd implied that they weren't. But then again, it seemed like his whole family was pretty involved with the hospital since the administrator had mentioned something about a wing carrying their name. Which meant they had to be pretty well off too. Not that it meant anything.

"That's good. Does Logan know Spanish as well?"

"No."

The answer was short, almost curt, and she decided that maybe she'd already outworn her welcome. "Well, I just wanted to check on Devon. Thanks for letting me know."

She got up to leave.

"Wait. Why don't we go ahead and set the time for our meeting? You're actually the last one on my list, so can you let me know when you're free?"

That was right. She'd come to give him those dates as well. But somehow it stung that she was the last one to meet with him, as if she were somehow the weakest link in the chain. Hadn't she wondered about that? Or were there more gaps in her self-confidence—thanks to Matt—than she'd realized?

Hell, you're reading too much into his words, Lucy.

She opened her phone and found the calendar app, where she'd marked the dates. "I have Friday of this week open and Tuesday of next week." She glanced up. "Do you need me to continue?"

He was looking at his phone as well. "Friday afternoon works for me. Do you want to meet here in my office?"

It was probably the best place, but then again, maybe it was better to meet on neutral ground, since being closed up in here with him was making her rather squirmy, even though he'd done nothing to make her feel that way. It was those damned butterflies. "How about the hospital café instead?"

"That's on the first floor, isn't it?"

"It is. You haven't been there yet?" There

were plenty of people who frequented the place. Maybe she wouldn't feel so out of sorts there. Because here in his office with his attention focused solely on her... Maybe it was still tied to the way he'd held that infant, his big hand cradling that tiny head in a way that said he'd done the same thing many, many times before.

The man could be the father of three for all she knew. But somehow she didn't think so. He didn't wear a ring and hadn't mentioned a wife or kids, but then again they hadn't talked much about their personal lives. He knew she had a sister, and she knew he had a brother and an ex-sister-in-law. And she certainly hadn't mentioned her broken engagement. Nor was she planning on it. But it was a good reminder that she shouldn't go daydreaming about anyone right now. Maybe in a year or two when the sting of rejection wasn't quite so strong. Actually she was feeling that same sting in being the last member of the team chosen and the last one contacted for that individual meeting.

"I haven't," Sam said. "It seems rather loud and noisy and—"

A knock at the door interrupted whatever he'd been about to say.

"Come in."

The door opened, and a slender woman with

well-manicured nails and an elegant air about her stood in the entry.

The woman's perfect brows arched. "So it is true. Why didn't you tell us you were back for good? I had to hear it from one of the nurses in Oncology. Not even Logan mentioned it. I thought your appearance at the gala was just a fluke or maybe you'd come to the city on business." Her attention swung to Lucy, and cool eyes very much like Sam's perused her from head to toe, taking in her scrubs and messy bun before she seemed to dismiss her. Lucy suddenly felt unkempt.

The woman's attention turned back to Sam. "I'm sorry. I didn't realize you were in a meeting."

"It's okay." He got up from the desk and went over and kissed the woman on the cheek, the act coming across as very strained. "The offer to work at the hospital came pretty suddenly. I would have gotten around to calling you, Mom. The fundraiser was just not the place for that kind of conversation."

Mom. This was Sam and Logan's mom? Her face was more youthful than Lucy would have expected.

And he hadn't "gotten around" to calling her? Lucy was in constant contact with both her parents and her sister, so it seemed totally alien to be in the same city as they were and not notify them. In fact, Lucy lived in the same Brooklyn neighborhood as her parents. And Bella still lived at home.

Whatever was between Sam and his mother wasn't something she wanted to witness so she stood. "Well, I'll let you two talk. I need to get back to my department anyway."

The woman looked at her again, peering closer as if trying to figure something out. "Aren't you going to introduce us, Samuel? Is this the friend you traveled to Uruguay with?"

There was a pause that stretched beyond the awkward stage. "No, Mom, Priscilla stayed in Uruguay. This is just someone I work with. Lucy Galeano, this is my mother, Biddie Grant."

"Nice to meet you." Lucy went over and clasped his mom's hand briefly, suddenly feeling an urgent need to get out of there. Even though she knew his words were true, being introduced as *just someone he worked with* had struck her oddly. Which meant whoever this Priscilla was, she'd been more than that. Or maybe she still was?

"You as well, Lucy. Are you a doctor too?"

"No, I'm a physical therapist."

"Ah… When I saw Logan after I did my reading in the children's wing and asked if it was true that you were actually back to stay, he mentioned it might be nice if we all met for dinner."

"Again, I'm sorry I didn't call you."

They were blocking the door and Lucy couldn't get out, but standing this close to them was about as uncomfortable as it got. She should have stayed in her seat, where there was at least some breathing room. These two were being so stilted with each other—as if they were total strangers. Not at all like her family, where hugging and laughing…or whatever the emotion du jour happened to be was the name of the game.

As if she sensed Lucy's discomfort, Biddie Grant said, "Well, Samuel, I'll let you get back to your meeting. Dinner on Friday, maybe?"

"Uh. I can't that day." He glanced Lucy's way.

She realized it was because he was supposed to meet with her. "Oh, that's okay. We can get together another time. Just let me know when you want to."

"Bring her with you, Samuel. You know Theresa always makes plenty of food."

"I don't think so," Sam said. "But we'll do it another time soon, Mom."

She's just someone I work with. For some reason tears pricked at the backs of Lucy's eyes, and she blinked rapidly to send them back to wherever they'd come from.

"Well, okay. But please do. Your father will want to visit with you too."

"I will. I'll call you."

Biddie sent her a smile that was as cool and elegant as the rest of her. "Well, it was nice meeting you, Lucy."

"You too."

With that, the woman turned, her low pumps clicking on the polished floor as she walked away.

What had she just witnessed? She tried again. "We really can meet another time. Your family should come first."

"Should it?" He seemed to realize how that sounded and continued. "No, it's fine. I'm sorry you had to witness that."

So he *was* aware of how awkward that had been.

"It's okay."

He smiled, looking world-weary all of a sudden. "It's really not. Let's not meet at the hospital. Do you mind if we go to a restaurant instead?"

"No, that's fine." But there was the matter of whoever Priscilla was. "But will it make it awkward for you and your…er, girlfriend?"

"My girlfriend? Oh, Priscilla. No. She was someone I was seeing, but that's over."

The image of a note on her pillow appeared in her mind's eye. She hoped he'd picked a better way of ending things than Matt had.

Lucy probably should not be going out to eat with him, especially with how she seemed to react whenever she was within ten feet of him. He obviously had no such problem. But if she tried to wiggle out of it now, he might wonder why. Or change his mind about her being on the team.

So she said, "Okay, dinner will be fine."

He nodded. "Pick a place and let me know where. I'm not as familiar with Manhattan as I used to be."

How long had he been in Uruguay? Long enough to have a relationship and travel there with whoever it was. Was that why he'd come back here? Because the relationship had failed? It also explained why he spoke Spanish well enough to know all of those curse words.

She couldn't ever imagine leaving her family or Brooklyn. She had a whole lifetime's worth of memories there. But Sam's personal life was none of her business. That was driven further home by the encounter with his mom. Had he been trying to emphasize that their meeting would be business only? No mixing of personal lives with work? Not that she would ever think otherwise.

So why was there a voice in the back of her head whispering something completely different? And why was it throwing out names of places that were quiet and intimate?

"All right. I'll do some searching and let you know what I come up with." And it would not be quiet or intimate.

"Sounds good." But the man was already back at his desk, sifting through papers and making it obvious that he was very busy. So she slid away on silent feet and wondered what the hell she'd gotten herself into.

The moment the door to his office closed, Sam tossed the papers aside and leaned back in his chair. His mom had picked a hell of a time to come say hi. He had a feeling he hadn't handled the introductions between her and Lucy very well, but he absolutely did not want his parents getting any ideas. Especially not after what Logan had gone through with Harper in the early days of their marriage.

Although Logan had never come out and said it, Sam was pretty sure his mom and dad had caused the rift that had resulted in their divorcing. It was one reason he was glad he and Priscilla had happened outside of the reach of their influence. That way he knew the breakup had been completely due to their own personalities and not for any other reason. In the end, they'd wanted different things out of life.

Priscilla, although she was a PA and still worked at the clinic, had gotten a side gig as a model once they'd moved to Uruguay. It was just before he'd overheard the conversation between her and her mother about how rich the Grant family was. She evidently wanted the swanky cars, posh life and media spotlight and realized she'd never get that in the medical field. Maybe it was why she'd started looking for modeling jobs.

Sam didn't care about his family's money. Not only didn't he care, he didn't want it—which was why he'd gotten rid of as much of it as he could. Actually his parents probably would have approved of his ex.

And Lucy? Would they have approved of her?

The thought of subjecting Lucy or any other woman to his parents made him cringe. Not that he and the physical therapist would ever be more than colleagues. Hopefully he'd learned his lesson as far as that went.

So why had he waited so long to have their meeting? He'd met with all of the other prospective teammates within days of that initial meeting, but he kept putting off Lucy's. Maybe because his mind kept playing over that spilled coffee and the amusing back-and-forth conversation they'd had? Maybe it had been that kick-to-the-gut attraction the second he heard that husky voice.

It was why he'd gone down to the physical therapy department the other day. He thought he could just wait until she was done with her patient and then go in and quickly give her the timeline he and the administrator had come up with for accepting patients. Except he'd gotten caught up in watching her use those puppets to reach a child who was scared and in pain. It had been heartwarming and very clever. It made him more sure than ever that she belonged on their team.

So he'd stood there and told himself he was observing, when it had gone far beyond that. And then she'd called him over, and he'd had to pry himself from that wall. Once she'd pointed out the mottling on her patient's back, the atmosphere had changed and he was no longer thinking about what she was doing and he was totally caught up in what needed to happen.

After that, he'd put off contacting her again. And again. Until she'd appeared in his office and asked how Devon was. And then there was no more getting out of it. The easy path would be to not include her on the team. But then he'd have to explain why, and the least professional thing he could do was exclude someone because he was worried about the way his body reacted when she was near.

If anything, watching her work should make him even more determined to include her, since she was obviously qualified and his observations had told him that she was willing to go above and beyond for her patients.

He should have just handed her the formal contract and sheaf of papers with the new department's information on it and been done with it, but that wasn't fair to her. And if he was going to head this thing, he needed to keep his personal feelings out of the arena when it came to his team. Something he'd never done very well when it came to his parents. They hated it when emotions took center stage, so he'd gone out of his way as a teen to make sure they did exactly that.

If his parents ever argued, Sam hadn't witnessed it. Nor did they show open affection to each other and only rarely to their kids. He had no idea how his sister was able to work for the family business. He knew he couldn't do it. Logan evidently couldn't either.

His mind came back to Lucy. Sam could admit there was an attraction there. He was pretty sure she'd felt it too in that conference room, although she'd never been anything but professional with him. And he had no idea why he'd suggested dinner out. Maybe because he'd been so relieved to get out of eating with his parents that he'd felt like celebrating. And she'd been sitting right there. Or maybe he just hadn't wanted another accidental meeting with his mom by meeting in the hospital cafeteria.

But whatever it was, he was going to have to make sure it didn't go beyond dinner. And it wouldn't. He had enough Grant blood in him to be able to appear cool, calm and collected when the situation called for it.

And this one did. Of that he had no doubt.

CHAPTER FOUR

THERE WAS A slip of paper on the desk in her cubicle written in what appeared to be a masculine scrawl. Lucy tensed, a sense of doom coming over her, before realizing there was no way her ex would have been anywhere near this place. He didn't like needles…or hospitals. Actually she'd met Matt through her sister, who'd been planning a wedding for one of his brothers. They'd gone out once and sprinted straight to bed. It had all happened so fast. Too fast, if she were honest with herself. But happen it had. The end of their relationship had happened with the same speed. As if he had problems with impulse control. Evidently so did she, since she'd been just as quick to jump into a relationship without weighing things first. It made her doubt her instincts. And normally she was pretty damned good at reading people.

But she wasn't going to go blindly into something like that ever again.

And the note? It was stupid to still react to them this way. But who wouldn't?

Well, obviously not her. Because a second ago, she'd been certain that note was going to be life-altering. She picked it up.

Just verifying tonight. Want to meet in the parking lot around seven? I don't know which restaurant you chose. Or if you've been too busy to think about it, I made a tentative reservation at Milo's, which came highly recommended from Logan. Text me if you already have a spot in mind, and I'll cancel the reservation.

It was from Sam and included his phone number this time, and she realized they hadn't exchanged them in his office the day his mom had come in. Which explained the note and why he'd had to come down to the PT department.

Damn. She'd completely forgotten he'd tasked her with choosing where they would eat tonight. Quiet and intimate? Wasn't that what she *hadn't* wanted? Well, Milo's had both of those things in spades.

She and Matt had been there several times, since as an architect he often met prospective clients there. And he'd even proposed to her on one of those dinner dates. Something else that seemed to come at lightning speed. Not something she liked to remember. But unless she wanted to lie and say she'd already picked out another place, it looked like she was stuck with it.

And she'd probably better at least acknowledge that she'd seen the note. So she typed his contact information into her phone and then answered him.

Seven is fine, as is Milo's. See you then.

Her thumb hovered over the Send button for several seconds before she finally pushed it. She then realized she'd forgotten to say who she was. But it should be pretty obvious right? Unless he was planning on taking other women to Milo's on other nights.

Who knew. He might be.

Her phone pinged seconds later. She swallowed and held it up to look. It was from Sam, but all that was there was a thumbs-up sign. Rather anticlimactic. But better than *Who is this?*

She could have simply responded, *Just someone you work with.*

That made her laugh. Maybe she shouldn't be glad that Sam and his ex had ended their relationship. But no matter how hard she tried to whisper those words to her brain, her heart kept kicking them right back out as untruths. And it was right. Because it wasn't true.

But even if she was, in fact, glad, it didn't mean that anything could come of them working together. Or that it should. She had hopefully learned her lesson about jumping into things sight unseen. And Sam had made it pretty plain that he wasn't interested, and that should've brought her a sense of relief. And it would, once she put any and all thoughts of office romances out of her head. She and Sam would be work colleagues. To hope for anything else was to invite disaster and ruin her chances of staying on the team.

Her next patient was here, so she threw herself into work and hoped beyond hope that everything went well tonight. And wasn't as awkward as she was imagining it was going to be.

Why had he thought this was going to be weird? Lucy was talking a mile a minute, and every other thing she said was as funny as hell. She'd just finished telling him a story about her dad calling the rest of their family to let them know he'd arrived at the restaurant where they were supposed to meet. But when he tried to follow the directions they gave him to their table, there was an elderly couple sitting there instead. It turned out that Gilberto Galeano had driven to a restaurant of the same name in a different neighborhood.

Sam couldn't think of a single funny story involving his mom and dad. Nor would they have found the humor in it if they'd found themselves in different restaurants in neighboring towns.

Priscilla had been beautiful and sexy, but her sense of humor was dark and often made him cringe when it was aimed at others. Whereas Lucy found humor in the lighter things in life and could laugh at herself with ease.

"So, did your dad drive back to Brooklyn?"

"No, we met him halfway at a different restaurant. So it all worked out in the end."

He pulled into a paid parking area a half block from Milo's, thankful his brother had warned him of the parking issues in this part of town. In fact, Sam didn't drive nearly as much as he had in Uruguay. Public transportation in NYC was great with subways, trains and even taxis all getting people where they needed to be.

"We'll need to walk a little bit to get there. Sorry about that."

Lucy kicked off the slides she'd paired with her dark-washed denim and tan short-sleeved jacket. "Not a problem."

She was going to walk barefoot? Why did that surprise him? It was the first time he'd actually seen her in clothes that weren't scrubs. She climbed out of the car before he could come around to let her out, looking perfectly at home with bare feet, her pink glittery polish winking at him in the sunlight that, even at seven, was still out. Spring in New York was pleasant for the most part. But there were hints of the heat that would soon attack the city when midsummer came.

They walked down the sidewalk with her swinging her shoes beside her. "So when is Devon's surgery?"

"It's actually on Saturday."

"Wow, surgery on a Saturday?"

"Greg wants to get this done and feels it's important enough that he's coming in on his day off."

"I am off, so I could come and observe. Will you be there?" As if thinking maybe that last question wasn't appropriate, she quickly added, "Not that it matters. And Greg might wonder if I suddenly show up."

"I was planning on being there, but even if I weren't, I have no doubt he would just think you were interested in it, since Devon is your patient too."

She smiled. "You remembered his name this time."

"I felt pretty silly not knowing who he was when you came to my office earlier in the week."

"I'm sure you have so many patients it's hard to keep them all straight."

"You seem to be able to."

"Not always. I do sometimes forget. I guess I have a little of my dad in me."

How easily she said that, as if being like her dad were of no consequence. If someone had told him he had some of his father in him, he would have probably been ready to throw down and fight. Because his dad and Lucy's were nothing alike.

But he also knew he probably had more of his dad in him than he liked to admit.

She turned so that she was walking backward when she asked, "Is there a timeline for when we accept that first patient?"

"You mean in the reanimation department?"

"Yes."

"Not yet. Todd wants to have a press release announcing the name of the new department. I think he hopes to garner additional funding to help with any unforeseen costs or price hikes. Microsurgery equipment is not cheap."

Lucy spun back to the front so that she was walking with him again. "Doesn't the hospital already do some microsurgery? I'm almost sure that they do. They could save costs by sharing equipment."

"Yes, but trying to manage equipment between two different floors could get dicey."

"I can see that. Do you think your father will help, like your family did the other hospital wing?" She stopped and bit her lip as if regretting her words. "I'm sorry. That's none of my business."

"It's okay. And no, he won't. I'm almost sure of it."

Her head jerked to the side to look at him, and Sam realized how that had sounded. "Let's just say my dad and I don't always see eye to eye."

She didn't say anything for a minute. "I kind of got that idea when your mom was in your office. I'm sorry. I can't imagine not having a good relationship with my mom and dad…or my sister, for that matter."

"You're lucky."

"I know I am." She glanced at him. "Do you think things with your parents will ever get better?" She added almost immediately, "Sorry *again*."

That made him laugh. "It's okay *again*. And I can't say that things will *never* get better, because obviously our new department is built on technology that no one thought would exist twenty years ago. So anything's possible."

"True. I guess there's always hope."

"There is. But there's a lot of bad water under that particular bridge."

Including his parents destroying his brother's marriage and his dad objecting to Sam leaving the country, even telling him not to bother coming back or expect any inheritance from him, that his grandfather's money would be all he would ever get.

Little had his father known that he neither wanted nor expected an inheritance. From anyone. If his dad was smart, he would leave his money to their sister, who was a shrewd businesswoman in her own right. Or to Logan, who would also do right by the money.

Was it wise to wish away any help his dad might want to give to the fledgling department?

Probably not, but gifts from Carter Grant normally came with strings attached. After he'd hired a lawyer to defend Sam after his arrest, his dad had then used that to try to strong-arm him into working for his company. Sam had refused. And things had been strained—to say the least—ever since then. Sam had put himself through medical school with scholarships and some student loans and had paid off those loans all on his own. He didn't want to be beholden to anyone, especially not his father. And when the time came to practice medicine, he'd chosen to work in Rochester rather than at Manhattan Memorial, although they'd wanted to keep him. At thirty-eight, Sam was pretty sure he was now as set in his ways as his father was. He didn't see either of them budging.

Lucy glanced again at him just as they reached the front entrance to Milo's. "Maybe it's time to clean up that water, then?"

Sam didn't have time to think about what that meant as someone from inside the restaurant opened the door and ushered them inside. He gave the hostess his name when she asked if he had a reservation. Within a minute they were being led through the dim recesses of the place.

He frowned. Maybe he should have asked Logan for a little more information when he'd given him the name of the restaurant. The fanciness of the place didn't faze him, but warm wood, leather and candlelight weren't what he'd expected either. "Have you been here before?"

"I have."

Lucy didn't expand on that statement, and he didn't press her for more information. But he was surprised that she'd want to come here with a work colleague, since it seemed more a place for romantic getaways.

He wasn't worried about the cost. At least not in terms of money. But he'd been feeling pretty damned good about this outing up until about a minute ago. Now all of those warm fuzzies that he'd allowed himself to feel were coming back to nip him in some places that were especially uncomfortable. Because he could easily get caught up in this atmosphere—in *her*— if he wasn't careful. She made being with her light and effortless. Just like her personality. No drama. No angst. She had a free-spirited air to her that made him want to stay close.

Priscilla had been serious and moody, always open with her feelings and emotions, and that had drawn him to her immediately. They were things he hadn't gotten at home, and their relationship had worked very well for a number of years. Until she seemed to want him to be more ambitious and to be more open to spending on luxurious living. She'd often hinted that he could easily be a hospital administrator or CEO with his people skills.

People skills? He had no idea what she was talking about because he was not an administrative type of person. He didn't see himself as having those talents or even wanting them. And money… Because he spent very little, he'd ended up with a bank account that was pretty padded even without the inheritance. Pri seemed to instinctively know that. And she sure as hell had found out that his grandfather had left him money.

So what had initially drawn him to her had ended up being the very things that drove them apart five years later. He'd needed someone more like he was—guarded and able to live a pretty independent existence without heavy displays of emotion. Priscilla had not been that.

Neither was *free-spirited and wildly funny*, the things that he liked about Lucy. And while neither woman was like the other one, the thing they had in common was that they were both in touch with their emotions and neither one of them was afraid of expressing them.

Well, Sam was. No, he took that back. He wasn't afraid of emotions in and of themselves. He just didn't let himself give in to them. Priscilla had wanted to hear the words, had wanted him to tell her he loved her on a regular basis, not realizing how much effort it took him to even say it once, let alone multiple times a day like she seemed to be able to do.

He really was like his parents. Damn.

He realized Lucy was staring at him in a

strange way. "What? I'm sorry—did you say something?"

She bobbed her head to the right, and he glanced over and realized a waiter was standing there pen and paper in hand. Oh, hell. How long had the man been waiting? And had he asked for drink orders, food orders...what?

"Sorry about that." He addressed Lucy, "What are you getting?"

"Water." She said it completely deadpan.

"Okay, thanks for all your help." He smiled. "I'll take a water and a whiskey. Preferably mixed."

Lucy laughed.

Yes, it was easy being with her. A little too easy. He was going to need to watch himself.

"Any appetizers?" The waiter still stood at the ready.

The problem was Sam hadn't even looked at a menu, which wasn't the case for Lucy, since hers was open in front of her. He couldn't believe he'd sat there staring into space for what probably seemed an eternity.

He glanced across the table. She shook her head.

"I think we're good," he said to the man. "But if you could give me a few more minutes to look at the menu I would appreciate it."

"Not a problem. I'll bring your drinks."

The man left, and Sam said, "Why didn't you say something?"

"I thought you'd eventually realize he was there."

"I normally would have." He didn't offer any more than that. Instead he changed the subject. "You said you've been here before. Any suggestions on what to order?"

"I like the eggplant."

Eggplant. Okay.

He'd never quite been able to get over the way that particular vegetable looked, although he did like the baba ghanoush he'd been tricked into trying at a dinner party in Uruguay. It was supposedly made of eggplant, and the dip had become one of his favorite dishes while he was there. Maybe he should give it a chance. "You mean as in eggplant parmesan?"

"You really haven't been here before, have you? Their specialty is risotto with eggplant and a special cheese. One that's not parmesan."

"Is that what you're getting?"

"I think so, yes. Although I've liked everything I've tried at Milo's."

The waiter came back about that time with their drinks and asked if they were ready. Sam nodded. "I think we are."

He waited for Lucy to place her order. She opted for a salad with her main dish, whereas when he ordered, he asked for a gnocchi soup with his risotto.

The waiter left, and Sam waited a minute or two before he said, "Do you want to wait and talk about the position after we eat, or are you happy to start now and continue on afterward?"

"Why don't we go ahead?"

"Okay. I don't have the official contract here in the restaurant, but I have a copy of it in the car. Even if you think the job is a good fit, make sure you look at the pay structure. HR will want to go over it with you."

She stared at him for a minute. "Um…will there be a cut in pay?"

"What? No, that's not what I meant. There will be an increase. I just meant it might not be as much as you were expecting."

"I actually didn't expect a pay increase at all, so that surprises me."

Sam smiled. "Are you saying you would have accepted the position even if there were a pay cut involved?"

"No. So don't get any bright ideas." She grinned at him.

He couldn't help but smile back. How did she do that, turn a serious conversation into something that was less weighty? "I wasn't thinking anything."

"That was pretty obvious a few minutes ago. You looked completely lost."

"Sorry."

"Don't worry about it. Thinking about the new department?"

His head tilted to the right. "You could put it that way. More like hoping we have the resources to do our patients justice."

"We will. You already have the talent in place. From what you said, all that is lacking is some specialized equipment. If necessary, we could even get that from a hospital that might be upgrading and be looking to get rid of its old stuff."

He wasn't sure how he felt about that. He was hoping to be cutting edge, but he saw her point. "Hopefully it will work out."

"And if it doesn't all come together as soon as you hope it will, what will you do? Leave?"

There was an expression on her face that he couldn't decipher.

He hadn't even thought about what he'd do. He'd assumed the hospital had already given a lot of thought to the needs of opening a new department. After all, they'd done it several times before. And his dad's money hadn't been necessary in all of those cases. In fact, contrary to

Lucy's assertion, his father was probably less likely to donate to a department that the son who'd given him so much grief was heading. Even though Sam would never admit that to anyone. Not even Lucy.

"I'm pretty sure the hospital has a plan in place for dealing with financing," he said. "I think that's why Todd has waited before announcing that change is coming. He probably wanted to be able to publicize the names of the team, hoping some of those names will generate some revenue for the new work."

"Okay. But don't expect my name to do that. I'm pretty much an unknown."

Sam didn't like the way she said that—as if what she brought to the table didn't amount to much—but the waiter had arrived, bringing Lucy's salad and Sam's soup and carefully placing them in front of them. He also brought an additional glass of water for Sam, who hadn't yet touched his glass of whiskey.

He did so now, bringing the tumbler to his lips and swallowing a healthy amount. It was the only drink he'd have tonight, and he wanted to savor it, since he probably wouldn't have more than that taste. He was driving, and he was no longer young and stupid. He'd done a lot of growing up since graduating from high school and medical school. His dad might even like the man he'd become if given the chance.

Sam just didn't want to give him that chance. He wasn't sure why, but right now wasn't the place to untangle the crazy web of his childhood.

"So what kinds of kids are you hoping for?"

"Excuse me?"

Her eyes widened. "I—I meant what kinds of kids are you hoping will come to the new department for help."

The words were said with care, and he realized he'd taken her question the wrong way. "I don't ever see the demand for these specialized surgeries taking the place of my regular practice, but you never know. The surgeries I've done until now have centered around the mouth. Cleft lips and palates and traumatic injuries to the tissues of those areas. I've performed surgeries at a clinic in Uruguay where more specialized procedures are done. Like grafting thigh muscles into the cheek as a way to repair impaired movement to areas damaged by other procedures or due to birth defects." He didn't know why, but he didn't want to mention that the clinic was one that had been part funded by his grandfather's inheritance.

"How about Moebius syndrome?"

He sat back in his seat, unable to hide his surprise. "Not many people know about Moebius."

"I actually worked with a patient with Moebius syndrome when I was a student. She was a sixteen-year-old girl. They were doing speech therapy with her, and there was talk of trying to do just what you spoke of. Microsurgery and grafting muscles and nerves to help repair the areas that had been damaged in utero."

"The so-called smile surgery?" Moebius developed in the womb and was due to damage to the sixth and sometimes seventh cranial nerve. The cause was thought to be an interruption in the supply of oxygen or due to drug use, although a genetic component couldn't be totally ruled out. Eye movement could be affected as well as parts of the face that helped relay emotion. The resultant paralysis of those muscles affected so many areas of a person's life. Whether it was nursing, eating, swallowing or speech. Part of Manhattan Memorial's new department would help those kinds of patients and others like them.

"Yes."

"Where was this?"

"Actually," she said, "it was here. The patient was having trouble getting cleared by her insurance company for the specialized surgery. And we didn't offer it here at the time."

"I know Mayo does it and a few of the other health-care giants. But if MMH's hopes are realized it means it will be within reach of other large teaching hospitals."

He picked up his spoon and ate a few bites of soup as Lucy did the same with her salad. The soup was wonderfully balanced with a creaminess that made him want more. But from what she'd said, their entree was going to be just as good.

Lucy paused and looked at him. "I think the program is going to be a success. As soon as I heard about it, I thought about that patient. I just never dreamed I'd be able to take part in something as important as this."

He smiled. "So I haven't scared you off yet?"

"No. I think it would take something huge to do that." She shrugged. "So if I'm hearing you correctly, I'll keep seeing my patients as per usual but will just jump in whenever a facial paralysis case comes in?"

"Yes. That's what all of us will agree to do. So we won't be dedicated entirely to the new department but will come together as a team whenever a new case comes in. We'll meet as a group and decide the best course of treatment that will encompass the patient as a whole, from pre-op preparation to the surgery to the aftercare and physical therapy. You will probably be their first and last stop," he said, "because you'll see the patient before we come up with a treatment plan and give us a baseline assessment. And then after the surgery you'll do their physical therapy and let us know how much change you see from where they started."

"Wow, I'm kind of surprised. I saw myself as handling the post-op physical therapy more than anything. But I really like your thinking as far as using PT as a measuring tool. I often think we're underutilized."

"I agree."

The waiter came with their entrees and set them in front of them, clearing away some of the other plates. "Would you like another whiskey, sir?"

"No, you can take the glass. I'd just like another water, please."

"Of course," the man said.

After he'd left she glanced at Sam. "You didn't finish your drink."

He gave a half shrug. "I'm driving."

"I'm sorry. I could have driven. Or we could have taken public transport."

"It's okay. I don't drink a whole lot anyway."

That was one good thing that his dad had instilled in him. Sam had never seen his dad drunk, although he and his mom did drink during social events. But they were both very disciplined and knew their limits. During his rebellious years, Sam had been reckless and had been lucky. But hopefully he was older and wiser nowadays.

Something touched his leg, and he blinked. Had Lucy just put her foot on him?

It had to be his damned imagination. There was no way she would do that, no matter how much of a free spirit she was.

But when it happened again, her foot sliding a bit higher, a spark of electricity went up his thigh and headed straight for his pleasure center. One that needed to stay asleep for the duration of this dinner. He moved his leg.

A few seconds later, her face turned blood red and she glanced under the table. "Oh, *Dios*! Was that your…your…?"

"My…leg? Why, yes. Yes, it was." He couldn't stop his slow smile when she couldn't seem to get the word out. And what could have become a very uncomfortable moment turned humorous. Especially when the horrified expression on her face made it clear she'd not done it on purpose. "I can put my leg back where it was, if you want, though."

"I swear I thought it was the table leg. Not a human leg. I hope you know I never would have—"

"I know. It's good to know, though, that you prefer table legs to real legs."

"I don't. I mean, I do..."

He had to rescue her. "I'm kidding, Luce. Don't think anything of it."

Because he would be doing enough thinking about it for the both of them. And not only about the smooth slide of her foot along his leg, but about his reasons for suddenly using the shortened version of her name.

Wasn't that how his relationship with Priscilla had begun? He'd shortened her name to Pri, and within a few days they were in bed together.

That couldn't happen here, though. He and Lucy could not wind up anywhere but in an exam room together.

Hell, that wasn't any better, because the images running through his head were now of them doing X-rated things in one of those rooms. Things where her foot on his leg was the least of his worries.

A half hour later, they found themselves back in Sam's car, and Lucy still couldn't believe she'd run her foot up his leg. *¡Dios!* Why was she becoming an absolute idiot when it came to Sam? Because the moment she reached for what she thought was the table leg a third time to find that it was no longer there, she'd taken a split second to process the possibilities and come up with the only probable explanation. And she'd wanted to die and slide under the table. Only he'd joked about it and given her that quirky smile and quickly put her at ease.

And then he'd called her Luce in that low silky voice of his, and it set all of her nerve endings on fire. They were still burning. Because she'd liked it. A little too much. The problem was she was pretty sure he had no idea he'd even done it. Kind of like the fact that she'd had no idea the "table" leg was actually his leg, probably because her shoe was on and she hadn't felt that it was denim rather than metal. She'd been about to do some very inappropriate things like run her foot all the way to the top of the table leg, something that had become a habit. It allowed her to stretch her leg in a way that no one could see.

But if she'd done it that third time, she was pretty sure she'd have discovered that the "table leg" gave way to something else entirely. And that was something there would be no coming back from.

"Anywhere you want to stop?" Sam put the

keys in the ignition and paused before starting the vehicle.

Maybe the nearest fire hydrant so she could cool herself off? If she were with any of her friends she wouldn't have hesitated to make that joke. But suddenly it didn't seem very funny. Because she really was having some weird and scorching thoughts, and she didn't know how to make them stop.

But she also didn't want what had happened in there to be the last memory he had of her: of her shoed foot climbing his leg in search of his...

No. She absolutely hadn't been in search of that.

"There's a little park around the corner. Do you have time to walk for a few minutes? I'm stuffed after that meal. And it's cool outside."

"I was just thinking along those lines myself."

She blinked. "You were?"

"Is that okay?"

"Yes. Yes, of course." Her nerves were stretched tighter than a violin right now. And doing anything with him, including walking, probably wasn't the smartest idea. But she really did want to get out of the car before she broke out in a sweat that might give her away.

He took the keys back out of the ignition and turned toward her. "Are you sure?"

Lucy mustered all the sincerity she could muster. "I am. I really could use some fresh air."

"Are you okay going to the park on foot so we don't have to go searching for another parking place?"

"Yes." She smiled for the first time since the debacle in the restaurant. "I was just thinking the same thing."

CHAPTER FIVE

IT WAS JUST after nine, and the temperatures were blessedly cool. Since it was Friday night, Manhattan was still teeming with people who were either out eating dinner or bar hopping, or just hanging out with friends. None of which described his current situation.

He was glad she'd suggested going for a walk, because he found he liked her company, even her funny way of apologizing for playing footsie with him.

"Which way is the park?"

When he'd lived in Manhattan with his parents, his life had been a whirlwind of school, sports and other activities. It was rare that Sam actually walked in a park. And as far as he knew, his parents never had.

"We'll turn right at the next corner."

This area looked vaguely familiar. He didn't think Milo's had been in existence when he was a kid, though. So it must have opened up after he'd left for Uruguay.

They turned right, and he saw a sign that sparked a memory. It was advertising an auto-repair shop with the funny slogan *Bad Wreck-ered? We can fix that*. He'd seen a sign very similar to that one on the day…

Then the park name came into view: Pirius Park. It was named after a figure in New York's history.

Hell. This was the park where the protest had been held when he was fifteen. The protest that had made him set a different course for his life and get his act together.

Rather than dread seeing it or it bringing up terrible memories, he saw it as a place of epipha-nies. Walking through the arched iron gateway, he saw it for what it currently was, without the angry students who were protesting too much homework. He'd almost forgotten what they'd been there for.

But now it was full of clipped hedges and groomed wood-chipped pathways, well lit and beautiful. In this section of the park swagged rows of twinkle lights hung over their heads and trees were draped in the same kind of lights. Not like Christmas decorations—it didn't have that vibe. It was more like a make-believe world where anything could happen. Like the changes in his life he'd made after his arrest? It was hard to believe that was over twenty years ago.

"I don't think I've ever been here at night," Sam said. "It's beautiful. And it's quieter than I would have expected it to be." Almost silent. Unlike it had been the day of the protest.

"Yes, it is."

They walked in silence for a few minutes, passing only one person as they moved deeper into the park. At the center of it, if he remembered right, would be a cleared square with some benches and an abstract fountain of some sort. The older man who'd fallen during the protest had been there to remember his wife who'd died the previous year. Pirius Park had been her favorite in all of Manhattan.

The memory rose unbidden and almost forgotten, but it was part of the reason why Sam had stopped to help him. He'd been looking for the picture of his wife that he'd dropped after being jostled. They'd found it, and Sam had walked the man a few feet to where the crowds had thinned out. That was when the police had stopped him.

So many years ago.

Lucy put a hand on his arm, stopping him. When he looked down at her there was a haunted sheen to her eyes. "I just want to say…this program is going to make a difference in so many lives, Sam."

"I hope so."

"I know it will." Her lips pressed tightly together as if holding back some strong emotion. "Remember the Moebius patient I told you about?"

He nodded, a sense of foreboding stealing over him. "You said you wished you knew whether or not she got the surgery." Was that what this was about? That it bothered her that she didn't know? Maybe that was why she'd been so anxious to know what happened with Devon. It was hard not knowing.

"Yes. I was talking to her one day, and she had this little dry-erase board that she would write messages on because it was hard to understand her most of the time. She turned her head to look around the room and then wrote *surgery?* with quick jerky movements. She pointed to it and then erased with a swipe of her hand. I got the feeling she didn't want anyone else to see." Lucy pressed her lips tightly together. "I was just a student and didn't know anything about whether or not she was going to be able to get it, so I told her to ask her doctor. But she shook her head and wrote the word again.

"I had to tell her I didn't know if she would get

the surgery or not, that I didn't make those decisions. I felt like a cad to even have to say it. And her eyes… *Dios*. Her face might not have been able to show emotion, but I saw what I thought was a pain so, so deep in those green eyes."

"I'm sorry, Luce." He brushed a strand of hair out of her eyes, feeling every bit of what she was saying.

"Do you know what she did then? She erased that word and wrote something else. She drew two circles. In the first one she wrote *surgery*. In the other circle she wrote *life*. She slowly drew a diagonal line through the first circle and then stared at the board for a long time. Then she put a line through the circle with the word *life*. I've never forgotten it, and I never want another patient to feel like that."

"I can't imagine. But we can't always give patients the outcome they want. Or that we want. Even in plastic surgery."

"I know. But I kept thinking it would be easier if that particular surgery were available at hospitals other than just the mega ones." She swallowed. "I've never told anyone about that experience before. I hope she found the help she needed."

"I do too. For what it's worth, I'm glad you told me." And he was. Not just because it would help him be more sensitive toward patients facing tough choices or who were fighting insurance companies or crippled with personal finance issues, but because it helped him understand Lucy even more. As if he hadn't already seen her concern when she'd dealt with Devon. He was positive that her Moebius patient had written those words to Lucy and Lucy alone because she'd seen what Sam saw in her. What probably a hundred other patients and their families saw in her: a compassion so deep that it gave them hope, made them want to trust.

His parents didn't have that. Neither did Priscilla. Not really. And it had Sam wanting to make confessions that were every bit as weighty as the one she'd just made about her patient. He struggled to keep bottled up how his upbringing had affected him or how much the sight of that old man searching for the picture of his dead wife had touched him.

He was able to bite back the words, but what he couldn't do was resist touching her cheek or saying, "You're pretty incredible—do you know that?"

"I'm not really."

"I'm not the only one who sees it. Devon's mom told me that he had another physical therapist at first who couldn't get him to cooperate. But you got through to him."

"It wasn't me. It was Quack."

Sam chuckled. "Okay, then. You *and* Quack are pretty incredible."

"Thank you." Their eyes met and held for several long seconds, and his thumb strayed from its perch and slowly traced the path from her cheek to her ear. Lucy made a soft sound deep in her throat before whispering his name.

His hands cupped her face. "So incredible."

Then his face lowered and his lips covered hers.

Dios. Lucy had been looking for relief from the heat that had been building inside of her, and she'd found it. Sam's lips were cool and soothing, and they touched hers like the softest snow. All of her cares melted away: The sadness over the patient she hadn't been able to comfort. The worries over not being good enough to be on Sam's team. All washed away by the press of his mouth to hers.

She couldn't stop herself from going up on tiptoe and winding her arms around his neck. *Santa Maria.* How had she not noticed how tall the man was? Lucy was not short by any means, but she had to stretch to reach him properly. And to kiss him properly.

And she loved it.

Loved that he'd known just what to say to make her feel better about herself. He hadn't given her some canned speech about how doctors were not responsible for what their patients felt or didn't feel. She knew that, though hearing it never helped.

What did help was that he knew that she did as much as she could for her patients. Not everyone recognized that, and he certainly hadn't gotten it from her bio. That only happened by getting to know a person on a level that went beyond team lead and team member. And yet they hadn't even started working together. How could that even be?

Her fingertips eased into his short hair, finding it oh, so soft, the strands shifting over her skin in a way that made it come to life. And oh, she never wanted this to end, wanted to stand here in the dark with him forever.

The sound of voices slid through her mind, and at first she thought it was just her inner monologue asking what she thought she was doing, until one of those voices laughed knowingly and then the sounds moved away.

Dios. Someone had seen them.

She pulled away, her arms slowly unwinding and falling back to her sides. "Someone was here," she whispered.

"Where?" His face was still close, his breath brushing over her cheeks in a way that made her close her eyes for a second. Then she forced them back open. No! They shouldn't be doing this. She'd already lectured herself on falling for someone again. Someone she barely knew.

She swallowed and took a step away, moving out from whatever spell he had cast over her. "It doesn't matter. They're gone now. But this isn't something we should be doing. We have to work together."

As if he, too, had come to his senses, he said nothing as she turned away, focusing her gaze on the lights behind them. They were still pretty, but they no longer held the magic that they had a few moments earlier.

Sam touched her shoulder, but she didn't turn around. "You're right, Lucy. I'm sorry. I never planned for that to happen."

"I know." She turned around. "Neither of us did. But I... I can't get involved with anyone right now. I'm just getting over a broken engagement, and things have been weird for the last five months since he left me."

There was a pause. "I'm sorry. I didn't know.

Priscilla and I ended a few months ago as well. Only I was the one who did the leaving."

"I bet you told her in person, though." She knew there was a bitter note to the words, but she couldn't help it.

"I did. I take it your ex didn't?"

"Nope. Left me a note that I found when I got home. Said he couldn't do it. All his things were gone, and I never saw him again. I even contacted the firm where he worked only to find he'd given notice, effective immediately."

Sam's brows came together. "Hell, I'm sorry, Lucy. But you're right. This is the wrong place and the wrong time...for both of us, it sounds like. I want to be honest, though. I don't think there will be a right place or time for me. It's not something I see myself doing again."

"I get it." For some reason, his admission made her feel better. She didn't have to worry about him wanting something more. Something she was too afraid to give at this point in her life. And it was the out she needed. And strangely enough, it helped her save face. He hadn't rejected her, specifically, and she hadn't rejected him. They'd rejected the idea of relationships.

And she was okay with that.

He tipped her chin up. "So we're good? I'd

hate to lose you from the team just because of my stupidity."

"You weren't stupid. Neither of us were. And no, I have no plans of withdrawing from the team. If you even tried to get rid of me, I might have to fight you."

"You would, would you?"

"Definitely."

He smiled and let his hand drop. "Then I'd better get you home before you change your mind."

She glanced at her watch, surprised to find it was after ten. "It's the witching hour for me, actually. I'm normally in bed by now."

"I didn't realize you had a curfew."

"That's the price of getting old."

He laughed. "I don't think you're quite there yet. But the last thing I want to do is keep a woman from her bed."

If they hadn't been interrupted, she might have asked him to share that bed with her. And that would have been an even bigger mistake. Because Lucy had always had a hard time separating sex from emotions. For her they tended to go hand in hand.

It was one thing to kiss the man. But go to bed with him? Look at what had happened with Matt. First to bed…then to living together. She couldn't do that again. And to let herself fall in love with someone who was about to lead the team she'd soon be involved with? That would be the biggest mistake she could imagine making. She made a pact with herself that she was going to stay out of Sam's arms. And whatever else she did, she was definitely going to stay out of his bed.

The press release went out four days after that kiss, and Todd sent a text to the team saying to get ready because the phones had been ringing nonstop ever since. With everyone from reporters to doctors from other hospitals who wanted to move to Manhattan Memorial to patients who wanted to be seen, there had been little time to think about anything but what was going on with the hospital.

Not that it didn't stop Sam from dissecting that kiss—every earth-shattering second of it. It was crazy and stupid, but he found it hard to not think about it at least once an hour.

He might've been thinking about it, but he hadn't talked to Lucy once since that walk in the park. He'd talked with most other members of the team, whose excitement was growing in the face of the media storm that was going on right now. Especially since it came almost on the heels of the hospital gala that'd happened right after he'd returned from Uruguay.

A knock sounded at his door. For a second he thought it might be Lucy, but the face that peered around the corner was definitely not feminine.

"Logan, come in."

His brother dropped into a chair. "Are you the reason why this place has gone crazy all of a sudden?"

Sam's brows lifted. "Would it surprise you?"

"Not at all." His brother laughed. "You always did like to stir the pot. Why should it be any different at MMH? Seriously, though, congratulations. I think this is going to be a great step for our hospital to take. I'm a little bummed not to be on the team, Not that we could ever work together without killing each other."

"If I remember right, you used to cover for me plenty of times with Mom and Dad."

"Speaking of Mom and Dad…"

Sam sank back in his chair. "Don't tell me she's now getting you to do her dirty work. I told her we'd have dinner soon. I just didn't commit. I'm not sure I'm up for seeing Dad yet."

"Not even for your niece or nephew?"

"You mean…" His eyes widened.

"We haven't told them yet."

Sam made a face. "I don't envy you that discussion."

"I'm not looking forward to it either. But Harper's about to the second trimester, and we can't put it off much longer. They don't even know we're officially back together."

"That's a tough one." He tried to imagine what would happen if he had to tell them that he and Lucy were a couple. Not that they ever would be. Right now that gave him a sense of relief that was larger than it should have been. And maybe he should be thanking Logan for keeping him grounded and making him even more certain of keeping his relationship status firmly in the *single and not ready to mingle* category.

"We are thinking of having a dinner in order to give them the news, and I wouldn't mind having a buffer there when we do. They made it pretty hard for Harper in the past. I'm not sure if Mom realizes just how terrible she was toward her. But we both agreed that we'll never let anyone step between us again."

"I'm happy for you. Really. I will say that what happened between you and Harper was one of the reasons I never brought Priscilla home to meet them. I didn't want them jinxing things. Moving to Uruguay seemed like a godsend at the time. But it turns out that sometimes things aren't meant to be, even when there's no one meddling."

Logan glanced at his face. "I'm sorry about that. I don't think I realized it was completely over. Are you sure? I mean, Harper and I thought we were done too, then…" His brother made a curving gesture over his midsection.

"I'm sure. It turned out Pri and I want completely different things out of life."

And yet sometimes even when people wanted the same things, they shouldn't be together. Like him and Lucy? Yes. Because it didn't change the fact that he couldn't—no, he didn't *want to*—tie himself emotionally to anyone other than his patients. And maybe he could with them because he knew it was for a limited time frame. After all, you could pretend to be someone you weren't for a short period of time. But for a lifetime? Well, it wouldn't work. At least not for him. He and Priscilla had tried that, but in the end, they just couldn't make themselves into something they weren't.

"I get it. But I'm still sorry. She seemed like a nice person."

"She is. And I only want good things for her."

Logan gave him an earnest look. "So…my real reason for coming. Do you think you can face Mom and Dad for a couple of hours while we tell them about the pregnancy? You can bring someone if you want, as kind of your own buffer."

"I don't think I'd want to put anyone through that, honestly. But I will come if it'll help."

"It will. I'll owe you big time."

"No, you won't. Consider it payback for all of those times we talked about that you covered for me. Do you have a day in mind?"

"Next week sometime? Maybe Tuesday or Wednesday?"

"At their place?"

Logan frowned at him. "You mean at our *childhood home*?"

That had come out wrong, and Sam hadn't meant it to sound like he resented his whole childhood. He didn't. He'd come to see that there were parts of it that were good and parts of it that were horrible. But one thing would never change. He loved Logan and Sarah, and he would always be in their corner. Sarah was already proving that she would run the company her way and refused to be a carbon copy of their dad. Sam bet Carter *loved* that.

"That's what I meant," he said.

"I'll see what Harper wants to do. Since it's our idea, she may want it at my place. I'm good with anything."

"I'll be happy to be there with you. Just let me know when. Maybe they'll turn out to be good grandparents. Stranger things have happened."

He didn't hold out a ton of hope for that, but diagnoses that looked hopeless sometimes found a way to turn themselves around.

"Thanks, Sam. Harper and I both appreciate it." He opened the door and turned to look back at him. "If it's worth anything, I really am glad you're home."

Sam smiled. "As strange as it sounds, I'm glad I'm home too."

Lucy's phone pinged as a text came through. She glanced up from the notes she'd been writing on a patient and looked at her phone which was on the far side of the desk in her cubicle.

Devon's surgery moved to tomorrow instead of Saturday due to pain in his back. Do you still want to observe?

Sam hadn't contacted her in almost a week, and she'd begun to wonder if he'd had second thoughts about her being on the team despite what he'd said after that kiss. The ride home had been a little awkward that night, but they'd seemed to part on good terms. But things could always change.

Just like people could always change, as she'd seen in her relationship with Matt. One minute he'd been a loving fiancé, then almost overnight, he'd wanted out of the relationship. So it stood to reason that Sam might have felt that kiss was a good enough reason to drop her from the team. And ultimately, it was his choice. Todd had made that clear when he'd spoken to the group, that just because their name appeared on a list didn't mean that list was written in stone and no one should take it personally if they were no longer included.

Lucy checked her schedule. She had a couple of appointments in the afternoon. It was a school day, so most of her work happened after the kids finished for the day. It was why she worked until six or seven when most of the other physical therapists got off at five.

She texted back.

a.m. or p.m.?

The little text box squiggled, letting her know he was writing a reply.

Eight a.m.

Okay, that was earlier than she normally got to work, but for Devon she would make it happen.

Yes, that works.

He replied with the number of the surgical suite, and that was that. There was no indication of whether or not he would be there too or if she'd be alone up there. It didn't matter. She was going either way, although if she were honest, it might be easier if he wasn't there. She would feel a little more comfortable, and her mind would be less on that damned kiss.

It always came down to that. Lucy somehow couldn't think about the man without that moment filtering back in. A moment that had lasted less than five minutes. She smiled. Actually that kiss had started way before their lips ever met. It had probably even begun when she'd mistaken his leg for part of the table. The seed had been planted then. It had germinated when they were joking about it. And the first blooms had opened when she'd talked about the heartache of her Moebius patient.

And then his lips had touched hers. And it had been wonderful and sweet and sexy and all the good things you associated with a kiss like that. Maybe it was even good that it had happened. Maybe they had gotten something out of their system that had been festering under the surface.

Festering. Ha! That was one way of looking

at it. In reality, it hadn't *needed* to happen. But she couldn't quite make herself sorry that it had. Lucy had semi-fantasized about him from the day of that first meeting in the conference room when he spoke to her in Spanish. So now that she'd kissed him and she no longer needed to wonder what it would be like, she should be over it. It was a most excellent kiss. And she would no longer have to mull over the possibilities in her head.

So if Sam was at that surgery, she would be fine. So would he. And hopefully Devon would come out of the procedure with the assurance that he could run and play like other kids without ever having to worry that doing so would endanger his mobility. It would be a win for everyone. And as long as she kept thinking like that, everything would be great.

Just great.

CHAPTER SIX

HE'D INVITED HER, so why was Sam surprised to
see her at eight o'clock sharp the next morning?
Maybe because she'd only arrived five seconds
before the procedure had started while he'd been
there since Devon had gotten to the hospital.

Greg Asbury was very good at what he did,
so Sam had no doubt that things would run well,
unless something unforeseen came along. And
he didn't see that happening.

There were several medical students already
here, so while he nodded to Lucy, he didn't motion for her to come down to the front and join
him. But she did anyway. He sensed her presence even before she actually sat in the chair,
and he wasn't sure how he felt about that.

"Sorry I'm late," she murmured. "The com-
muter train was running behind."

Interesting. Why didn't he know she took the
train? He couldn't remember if she'd actually
told him where she lived.

He wasn't sure what that said about him that he could kiss a woman without knowing much about her.

Except he did. He'd read her eyes when she told him about her patient and those word bubbles on the white board, just like she'd read that young woman's eyes when she wrote them.

And that kiss had been…

Well, he hadn't quite found an adjective that would describe it. Or maybe he was just afraid to look for one.

No, that wasn't it at all.

So why hadn't *he* heard the people she said were there when he'd been kissing her? Had he been that caught up in what was going on that he'd blocked everything else out? Or had Lucy made them up as a way of getting out of telling him the truth—that she hadn't liked kissing him?

The hell she hadn't. Those fingertips pressed against his scalp told a different story. The way she'd held him against her as if afraid he would simply disappear. Those were the acts of someone who liked what was happening.

But it wasn't going to happen here. Or anywhere else for that matter. And he needed to keep his mind on Devon's surgery, or he would miss that too.

Greg kept up a running commentary as he went through each step. Opening the skin, going through the muscles, checking the vertebrae with methodical accuracy.

It looked to be intact and capable of protecting the cord once they were able to separate it from the structures holding it in place. That was getting ready to happen.

The neurosurgeon had told the family the mottling should subside once the spinal cord was no longer attached, although Devon would now have a scar in its place.

"Getting ready to free the cord."

Everyone held their breath as complete silence enveloped the room. Greg didn't play music while operating, unlike Sam, who liked to have the soft sounds of instrumental jazz in his surgical suite. Five seconds went by. Ten. Then Greg stood up straight and glanced up at the observation room and gave a thumbs-up. "It's free. And it looks good. This boy will be able to go back to playing T-ball and should have a normal life."

Excited murmurs went through the room as Greg went back to work finishing up the surgery. Sam felt a hand squeeze his for a single second, and then it was gone. Almost before he'd had a chance to register its presence. And when he looked down at Lucy, she acted like nothing had happened. Had he just imagined it?

No way. He knew her touch, although he had no idea how or why. But he liked that even after what had happened, she wasn't afraid to squeeze his hand in a friendly way. Maybe because that was what they had become. Friends? Or if they weren't exactly there yet, they were hopefully circling around that point looking for a place to land. Because friendship with her would be… better than the alternative, which was aloof colleagues who were there for the job and not much else.

Although hopefully the team would become close enough to be able to bat around ideas without involving egos or a sense of turf. They all needed to work together as one unit.

Kind of like that kiss? Where he and Lucy had become fused into one being?

Oh, hell.

He needed to stop this. Lucy stood, and he followed her up.

"I can't believe it was that simple. Not that it was really. But it was so fast. All that worry and now it's almost over. Once he heals, he'll be able to go on with his life." She sucked in a breath. "I'm hoping that for any and all patients who come through the facial-reanimation program too."

"There are a lot of us who think the same thing. Do you want to go talk to Greg?"

"I do. You?"

"I'd planned on it."

They went down and met Greg as he was coming out of the room. He'd already stripped off his gloves and hat, but his booties were still on his feet.

"Nice work," Sam said.

"Thanks. It's always good when it turns out to be pretty much as you imagined it would be. Nothing complicated. Thankfully the cord itself wasn't tangled up with the skin cells. We just need to let him heal and hope there are no postop complications."

"You'll keep us updated?"

Greg glanced from him to Lucy. Sam gave a silent curse. He hadn't meant to make him and Lucy sound like a unit, but evidently the neurosurgeon had heard differently.

Fused. Wasn't that the term Sam had just used in his head?

Lucy smiled. "Thankfully Sam was down in PT the day Devon's shirt came off, revealing the mark."

Good save, Luce.

"Well, I'm glad you both saw it. Because even though the nerve cells hadn't grown through the skin, the skin could have become a stricture that could have later tightened or pulled against the cord, causing a tremendous amount of damage. The pain he felt in his back this last week gave evidence to that, as did the fact that the nerves in his feet were being affected."

"Which is why his mom noticed him tripping?"

"Exactly." Greg smiled at both of them. "I'd better head for the waiting room and let Mom know that things went well. See you both around. I'm hoping that our new department will start hopping soon."

"I have no doubt it will."

Greg stopped and turned to Lucy. "Oh, are you responsible for the dog puppet that Devon brought with him to the hospital?"

"You mean Spot?"

"Yes. That's the one."

Lucy looked a little unsure. "Yes, but I always sanitize them between patients, so…"

"No, it's not about that. He almost refused to have the surgery if Spot couldn't be there with him. I had to reassure him that the puppy would be right beside him when he woke up."

"Yikes. Sorry."

"Don't be. I think it's nice. And I already read the recovery team the riot act and told them to make sure the hound is there when he wakes up. I don't want a child calling me a liar." He laughed. "Okay, see you two later."

Greg left to do what he needed to do, leaving the two of them standing there. Sam smiled. "You and those puppets."

"What? The kids love them."

"That part is obvious." He paused. "You don't have patients this morning?"

"Not until after school. But it's not worth traveling back to Brooklyn only to have to turn around and come back in a few hours."

He frowned. "I'm sorry. I didn't realize you came in specifically for the surgery."

"Don't be sorry. I wouldn't have it any other way. I'll just grab some breakfast."

He thought for a minute. "Are you interested in making your breakfast a working one? I have a patient I'd like you to see, and then I could use some help running through a mock case file. When we do actually start getting more patients, I'd like to have a step-by-step chart that starts with the patient's referral and follows them all the way through to completion. It's hard to get all of us together, since we all work different schedules. I'll still get the other team members' input on it, but if you have time and wouldn't mind being a sounding board…"

And if she didn't want to? Then he'd have to respect her decision and would handle it on his own. Todd couldn't help him because he wasn't actually a doctor and some of the logistics would be out of his realm of expertise.

"Sure. It'll keep me from twiddling my thumbs down in my cubicle."

His brows went up. He wasn't sure how he felt about barely making it above the level of twiddling thumbs, but at this point he'd take what he could get. "Are you good seeing the patient first?"

"Yep."

Together they walked down the hallway. Abby Garner needed one of the surgeries that would soon be done on a regular basis at the hospital. So as they walked he gave Lucy a rundown on what they were looking at. "How much do you know about nerve transplantation?"

"Some, from my studies in kinesiology."

"This patient is an adult, but she fits the bill of what we are looking to do in kids. Her facial nerve was damaged during surgery for a tumor on one of her salivary glands a few months ago. While the surgeon was hoping the function would come back as she healed, that's not been the case. And there's a window of about two years for us to do a masseter nerve–to–facial nerve transfer."

"Masseter nerve involves chewing, correct?"

"It does. With Abby, we're hoping to take one branch of the masseter nerve and graft it onto the part of the facial nerve that involves smiling."

"Ah, the smile surgery that we talked about earlier."

They stopped in front of the door. "Yes, exactly. I know you deal with children, but I'd like her to go through PT with you once she's a few weeks out of surgery, since you're on the team. It takes six months or so for us to really get a good picture of how successful the surgery will be. We'll be getting some advice from a sister hospital along the way."

"I'm excited to get started."

They went into the room. The patient was a twenty-one-year-old woman. Sam introduced them and then watched as Lucy talked to her and asked to examine her facial muscles.

Abby gave her permission, and Lucy went through a wide range of exercises designed to see where she stood as far as her facial muscles went. In fact, he was surprised at the way she deftly identified the muscles for each facial movement and decided which ones worked normally and which ones showed signs of impairment.

"Will you be able to fix it?" Abby spoke very slowly, each word seeming to take an enormous effort.

Lucy glanced at Sam, as if waiting for him to talk. He explained the procedure and what he hoped it would accomplish. "It'll require some patience on your part because nerves take a long time to heal and start firing again."

The patient nodded and pointed at Lucy rather than trying to talk again.

"Yes, I can help do your physical therapy, if you think we'd be a good match."

"Y-yes."

Sam gave the patient's shoulder a soft squeeze. "We'll need to go through your insurance company and get the surgery approved. Once that's done, we can schedule you and hopefully restore most of the function you've lost."

Abby nodded, but when he glanced at Lucy he saw she was frowning. Did she disagree with something he'd said?

Once they finished here, he'd ask her.

They spent a few more minutes with Sam explaining the procedure in more detail, using a video demonstration of how the transplant would be done. And then they said goodbye.

"I hope to see you in PT in the not-so-distant future." Lucy gave her a soft smile that made his stomach clench. She was good with her patients in a way that he never would be. He was much more direct, much more matter of fact. But Lucy dealt in hope. In hard work and effort. And in the PT world, all of that probably did make a difference. Hopefully it would for Abby and all of their future patients.

As they left the room, he glanced at her. "What's on your mind?"

She didn't ask what he was talking about. "What if insurance denies her the surgery?"

"There's always that chance. But we won't know if we don't try."

She shook her head. "She needs this surgery. I've never understood how anyone can say no. Isn't there a way around it?"

Was she thinking about the patient she'd mentioned from years earlier?

"There's always the ability to pay out of pocket, but most people can't afford it. But MMH is hoping to have grant money that will help fill in some of those gaps. And I'll be donating some of my time on some of these cases where we know finances are an issue."

She seemed to relax. "That makes me feel better."

"Let's just take it one step at a time and see where things go." He glanced at her. "Are you still up for helping me on the project? You can see from meeting Abby that we need to have a set of guidelines in place…and dealing with insurance companies is part of that process."

"Yes. I'd love to have a say in it. But can I run by the cafeteria first and grab a bite to eat?"

"Of course. Sorry—I should have thought of that."

She smiled, her nose crinkling. "Not a problem. Do you want me to bring you something from the cafeteria?"

"Maybe just a coffee?"

"Okay." She started to walk away before turning back to him. "Cream? Sugar?"

"One of each, if they have it."

"Got it. See you in a few." She walked away, and the gentle sway of her hips brought his attention to the pattern of her scrub top. It was the same parrot one she'd worn a couple of times. She must've really liked it.

He should too, because it bore the reminder to *repeat after me*. Something he'd been doing for the last week. Repeating over and over that he shouldn't kiss her again. No matter how much he might want to.

* * *

Lucy asked for her food to be put into a bag to make it easier to carry upstairs. Shoving their coffees into a drink carrier, she managed to balance the bagged breakfast on top of it and headed to the elevators.

Sam's brother, Logan, happened to be there as well and smiled when he saw her, glancing at her hands. "You must really like coffee."

"Actually one of them is for… Sam." She hesitated before adding his name. Then hurried to explain. "He's trying to make a protocol for our eventual facial-reanimation patients and asked for some input on it."

"I see."

Had her explanation made things better or worse? She wasn't sure, but if she kept trying to explain over and over she was going to come across as being in too much of a hurry to explain away something that had very little significance. Unless she made it seem like it did.

And that was the last thing she wanted to do. So she just let it stand. Thankfully the door opened, and they both got on.

He pushed the button for the fourth floor, even though the neonatal department was housed within the maternity ward. But when she reached to push the floor for him, he shook his head. "I'm headed to Sam's office too. But I just need to tell him something quick, then I'll be on my way."

"Oh, don't hurry on account of me, okay? Sam and I can always do this later."

"Nope. He doesn't even know I was coming. I just wanted to give him the details on our dinner with our parents."

Oh, so he was going to have dinner with them after all? Sam had made it seem like he and his parents didn't get along all that well. Actually, she'd gotten that impression when his mom was at his office trying to get him to commit to coming over for dinner. Something he'd never actually done while she was standing there. Instead he'd put her off, saying she would call him.

"I'm glad to hear they were able to nail down a date."

Logan blinked. "A date?"

Ugh, he had no idea what she was talking about, and Lucy didn't really want to explain that this wasn't the first time that she'd been in Sam's office. Or make it sound like they'd discussed his personal life. They hadn't. Not really. She'd simply happened to be there during a very uncomfortable encounter between the two.

"Your mom happened to come by while Sam and I were discussing the new department."

That was the closest she wanted to come to admitting that she knew anything about them. But the fact that she kept calling him Sam rather than Dr. Grant might be something he looked askance at too.

"Ahh, yes, he told me about that."

He had? What exactly had he said?

She couldn't think of anything to say, so chose to say nothing at all.

Logan glanced at her and then said, "He said she wanted him to come over for dinner and he hadn't given her a date. So Harper and I invited Sam to come over when our parents are going to be there. We figured it would make things easier on everyone. Harper is expecting a baby. And we really could use Sam there as a buffer. Or as a witness." He grinned in a way that looked very much like his brother's smile.

"Oh! Congratulations on the baby. I didn't know."

"Not everyone does. Thankfully Sam was gracious enough to agree to come. I just need to confirm the date and time. It'll only take a minute."

The elevator doors opened, and she stepped off, juggling the coffees and the bag as she pulled one of the hot drinks from the carrier.

"I'll let you go in there first. This is his coffee, if you don't mind giving it to him."

"You don't have to wait outside."

"It's okay. I'd prefer it that way."

Logan looked a little bit confused, but he took the proffered cup. Lucy couldn't blame him. She was turning this into something weird, but she couldn't figure out a way to go back and undo anything she'd said. Not that she'd actually said anything that made it sound like they were meeting for personal reasons.

They weren't.

But he doubted that Sam had told his brother about that kiss either. So the last thing she wanted to do was be the one who let the cat out of the bag. Talk about making a big deal out of nothing. She was pretty sure she'd used those exact words with Sam and told him it was *not* a big deal.

Without saying anything else, she found the little waiting room that she'd sat in the day she'd exited the elevator and seen Sam cradling that baby.

Lucy dropped into a chair and put her breakfast on the seat next to her and bent over to cradle her own head in her hands. *Dios*. Why was she acting guilty about meeting him in his office?

Was it that she *felt* guilty? Because of that kiss?

She hoped not, because he'd made it clear that he wanted to put that behind them. And the fact that he'd asked her to help him to construct a template for future patients said he'd been able to do just that: put the kiss behind him. So why was she having a heck of a time doing the same? She had no idea, but she'd better put things back on a normal track, or Sam was going to figure it out and things would become super awkward between them. And she didn't want that.

A few seconds later, Logan went by and gave her a wave. "See? Done. He's all yours."

Lucy knew the man had no idea how that had just sounded. At least to her. All because of those crazy thoughts she kept having.

So she stood and went to his door, which was thankfully standing open, because she wasn't sure how she was going to knock on his door with her hands full.

Poking her head in, she saw he was looking at something on his phone. "Are you ready for me?"

He shut whatever app it was and held up his coffee. "Thanks for this. But you didn't have to stay in the waiting area. Logan didn't stay long."

"I know, but I kind of…" She crinkled her nose. "I kind of gave it away that your mom was here and that you hadn't given her a date for dinner."

He smiled. "Logan already knew about that. I told him. No big deal. Harper is expecting a baby, and he wanted me there when they told my parents."

"That's what he said. So you're going to be an uncle. Congratulations."

"Thanks. Better him than me, though."

She tilted her head. "You don't mean that. I saw you holding that baby the first day I came up here. You looked like a natural."

"That's only because I could hand her back over to her real mom."

"But surely someday…" Why was she interrogating him? Hadn't she gotten a kind of sick feeling in the pit of her stomach about babies after Matt had left? Maybe it was the same with Sam, since he'd broken up with his girlfriend.

"I think my dad will be a lot happier that Logan and Harper are the ones making them grandparents than the alternative."

"I'm sure he would be just as happy if it were you."

He looked at her for a minute. "You don't know my father. Well, anyway, shall we get started?"

"Yes. Of course."

She found her seat and saw that he had a big blank pad of paper on his desk with a permanent marker laid across the top of it.

Then he stood and picked up his coffee. "This will be easier if we're on the same side of the desk, so is it okay if I join you?"

"Of course." Lucy obviously hadn't thought this out clearly. Somehow she'd been picturing constructing a PowerPoint presentation, with him sitting on one side of the desk and her on the other.

As he sat in the chair next to her, the same warm scent of timber and earthy forest floors enveloped her, just as it had when they'd been in the observation room watching Devon's surgery. It was the same scent that had also curled around her senses when they'd kissed in that park a week ago.

And as it had this morning, it brought back memories that she'd been trying so hard to bury. Trying so hard to put behind her, like she had Matt. But for some reason this was proving much harder to do. But she needed to keep working at it. Maybe this meeting would give her a chance to do exactly that.

She tried to make a light moment of it. "Somehow I thought this was going to be a little more high-tech than pad and paper."

His head tilted. "Does that bother you? I always work better when I can actually write the words out rather than typing them on an app."

"I was thinking more along the lines of a PowerPoint."

He smiled. "I'm not quite that computer literate."

"Really?" She did presentations all the time. It was a good teaching tool for her patients, and several times she'd sent parents home with a flash drive of instructions and suggestions for exercises. "I can write one up later, if you want."

"Are you serious? That would be great for when the team meets next. If you don't mind manning the computer as I talk my way through it."

She shrugged. "I would be happy to."

"I think it'll make Todd happy too. He's been after me to get him something in computer form. I was afraid I was going to end up sending him a big piece of paper with a graph drawn on it with lines leading here, there and everywhere."

Lucy crossed her legs, and her foot accidentally bumped against his shin. Memories of her foot trailing up his leg at the restaurant made her stutter out an apology. "Sorry. That was an accident, I swear."

A laugh came from the man next to her. "You have your share of accidents, don't you?"

She bit her lip. "Evidently I'm a magnet for them. Good thing I didn't go into neurosurgery."

His hand covered hers for a second. "I was kidding, Luce. I have no doubt that if you'd gone into neurosurgery, you would be as successful at that as you are at physical therapy."

A sense of relief went over her. She had had a lot of little slip ups when he was around. It had to be nerves. But at least he wasn't taking it as some kind of shortcoming on her part. "Thanks."

They got down to business, with both of them throwing out ideas and trying to decide where each step would fit on their chart. The insurance part of it was the most complicated because they had no doubt that some of those companies would automatically throw the procedures out, citing them as experimental, even though almost all of them had been around for a while in some form or another. So additional steps for the appeals process would need to be taken into account.

"Okay." Sam tore off the sheet they'd been working on. It was a mess of writing and scratch outs by now, and he set it on the desk next to a new clean sheet of paper. There were three other discards that were beneath that one. "Let's try to make some sense out of this."

"You're right. I have no idea how we would get this onto a PowerPoint without graphing it out on paper first."

He looked at her as if feigning surprise. "I think you're the first person who has ever spotted the genius behind my madness."

"I never used the word *genius*."

"But you know it's true, right?"

She bumped shoulders with him. "It's true that I never used the word *genius*."

The bump was returned. "Just give it time. You will."

This was really nice. Now that her nerves had settled down, they'd actually gotten quite a bit done. And she was surprised to find that they worked well together, even though they both saw things from a different point of view. Sam was definitely more task-oriented and was all about getting the job done, while Lucy took into account a patient's emotional state and was more about giving them time to process things. Of course, a lot of Sam's patients needed things to happen quickly, while her job saw recovery as more of a process that took time. But maybe that's what made it work so well. They complemented each other.

They hashed through the process one more time, and this time the sheet of paper only had one thing scratched through and one arrow that moved something to a different location.

Lucy glanced at her watch, surprised to find that it was almost one o'clock. "I have a patient coming in about an hour, so I probably need to get ready for her."

Sam stretched his arms up and over his head, giving a groan. "And I probably need to get out of this chair before I become glued to it." He glanced at the paper. "But I'm happy with this. You?"

"I think it's good. But I do think it would be good to have some more input on it."

He nodded. "Were you serious about putting it into PowerPoint form? Or can you not even figure out how to organize it?"

"I think we've done a good job of doing that. All that's needed is to plug it into the program. It's not that hard. I can work on it later this evening."

"No, don't. Give yourself a break. If you could get it to me by next Friday that would be soon enough. I can let Todd know it's coming."

"I'll definitely get it to you before then. How about Tuesday afternoon? We can go over it together, and you can make sure it looks how you expect it to."

"I am tied up the rest of the week with meetings. And Tuesday…" He seemed to think for a minute. "Well, that's the night Logan asked me to come over for dinner while they tell my parents. So maybe afterward…? I've been racking my brain for a way to get out of there within a two-hour time frame."

He sighed again. "But then that would mean that you'd have to sit around and twiddle your thumbs until I'm done. And we both know how much you like doing that."

She laughed, remembering their early conversation.

"I could wait in the car and serve as the getaway driver." A thought occurred to her. "Or I could come with you, if you don't think Logan and Harper would mind. But then again, that's kind of a personal time for them, and as an outsider—"

"I'm pretty damned sure they wouldn't mind." Sam seemed to leap on her idea with lightning speed. Had he already been thinking along these lines?

But whatever it was, it was too late for her to take back the idea. "Are you sure?"

"If you really don't mind? It would lend weight

to the idea that I really do have a project that has a deadline. And I really don't want to get into a heated discussion with my dad, which seems to always happen when we're together."

"That bad, huh?" She'd never had to be someone's exit excuse before.

"It could be, although it's been a long time since I've had any kind of lengthy discussion with him. Then again, it might be fine. But I'd rather dip my toes into the water and then wade a little deeper each time I see him."

Ooh, she was no longer so sure her idea was a good one. Hadn't his mom already asked if Lucy was the one he'd gone to Uruguay with? But she saw that really he was struggling with going, and she'd been the one to suggest that he work on cleaning up the "bad water" that had gone under their bridge. So to renege on her offer didn't feel right either, since it was obvious he wanted to support Logan and Harper. "We don't have to pretend to be a couple, right?"

He seemed taken aback. "I would never ask you to do that."

"Sorry—I think I phrased that badly. I just don't want them to get the wrong idea about us."

"Logan knows we're just colleagues, and I'll let him know ahead of time. He said he wanted to use me as a buffer between them and Dad and even suggested I take a plus-one as a buffer for myself. I didn't think I needed one, but…maybe having an 'outsider' isn't such a bad idea. My parents are all about public image. And this is important to Logan and Harper. They've been through a lot. And I…"

"And you don't want to leave things with your dad for longer than necessary."

"How did you know?"

"It was more a suggestion than guessing your motives behind going." She shrugged. "None of us knows how much time we have on this earth, and I believe we should be at peace with everyone we can be. Unless there's been abuse or some other reason."

"No, nothing like that. As much as I hate to admit it, I do want to make my peace with him. If it's possible. And if it's not, I want to walk away knowing that I tried."

She smiled. "Exactly, Sam. What time are you supposed to be there?"

"Seven. They'll have dinner. Nothing fancy. No catering or employees."

Her eyes widened. "Why am I thinking that the opposite is the norm when it comes to your parents?"

"Because it is. But Harper wants to set a new tone with them and wants some boundaries set firmly in place when it comes to protecting her and Logan's relationship and for when the baby comes. But they'll do that after I leave. I already told Logan I probably wouldn't stay longer than dinner, and that works out for them as well. If things fall apart, then my parents will probably be leaving early as well."

"Oh, wow. I hope that's not the case."

"I hope not either. Thanks for offering to come. I'll try to make sure you're not subjected to anything that makes you uncomfortable. Just nudge me under the table."

"Do you want me to do that with my foot or..."

Sam laughed right on cue, and she was glad that she could make him feel a little bit better about something that was obviously hard for him. "It depends whether it's *my* leg or the table leg."

"Why, your leg, of course."

With that, they wound things up, and Sam pulled the sheet of paper off of the block and folded it before handing it to her. "Don't you want a copy of that first?" she asked.

"I trust you."

She sure hoped he wasn't misguided in that trust. And she hoped that when they were at Logan's house that she wasn't tempted to step in and play a part she had no business playing: that of Sam's *significant* other.

Because that wasn't what she was. And it wasn't what either of them wanted.

So why was she suddenly so very tempted to do exactly that?

CHAPTER SEVEN

OH, HELL, WHY ON earth had he agreed to go to Logan's tonight? And why was Lucy letting him drag her along with him? It really wasn't fair of him to expect her to come, even though she'd been the one to offer. But he couldn't imagine she was looking forward to it any more than he was. Although she'd texted him this morning and said that she'd finished the presentation and they could go over it after leaving the party.

Party? He doubted very much that tonight would be very festive, although he genuinely hoped that his mom and dad didn't make Harper sorry that she and Logan invited them into this part of their lives.

At least he could look forward to seeing what Lucy had accomplished with all their chicken scratch and know that the next big hurdle toward the official opening of the new department was going to be behind them. Todd had shared that they already had a couple of grants lined up that would pay for most of the new pieces of equipment that they would need. And they had arranged for a huge teaching hospital to fly over a few members of their own facial-reanimation team to come have a Q&A. Thankfully the center didn't see them as competition but rather a way to relieve their own workload that found patients stuck with hefty wait times.

Another few months and they should be where they needed to be. They might even be able to take a patient or two before that if the stars lined up right.

He glanced in the bathroom mirror, giving his hair a quick comb-through, trying to see what his dad would see when he looked at him. They'd barely spoken at the gala.

Sam already had some gray showing through his hair, and there were lines in his face that hadn't been there when he'd left for Uruguay two years ago. He'd also let some scruff grow on his face, which his dad had never been a fan of. On anyone.

But regardless of whether or not his dad approved of the way he looked or lived his life, Lucy was right. It was time. If things could be made right, he wanted to do so now before it was too late. Their sister couldn't make it tonight—she was working late—but promised to try to get together with the siblings another time. Sam wasn't worried about Sarah. They'd always gotten along.

He set the comb down and shrugged his way into the blue button-down shirt he'd planned on wearing with his jeans.

Lucy expected to meet him at the hospital at six thirty; she'd arranged to have her last patient come in a little earlier than normal so that she'd be done in time. He halfway hoped she'd be dressed in her parrot scrub top. It was his favorite.

And why did he even have a favorite piece of clothing for her?

It didn't matter. He'd already figured out how to introduce her. She was a colleague on his team, and they were working on a presentation that needed to be done by tomorrow morning. They'd decided to kill two birds with one stone, and Logan inviting him to dinner had been perfect timing. He didn't really care if they bought the explanation or not. It was true enough, and if they chose to believe something else? Not his problem.

But then again, he'd promised Lucy that he'd make sure no one thought they were a couple, so he needed to smack down any stray questions or comments that his mom or dad made that looked like they were leaning in that direction. There was no need to put her in the middle of anything.

He went out to where he'd parked his car and was able to make it to the hospital by six thirty sharp. Lucy was already waiting out front and slid into the passenger seat. She wasn't wearing her parrot scrubs but rather was dressed in a white ribbed tank top over a flared black skirt. She looked cool and comfortable yet elegant. She glanced at him, her lips twisting as if needing to tell him something but not sure how. Maybe she was going to back out on him.

"Second thoughts?" he asked.

"Not about coming tonight, but there's been a slight hiccup. I know you wanted to work on the presentation tonight. But after I got to MMH tonight, I remembered that I need to move my car. The street sweepers will be there in the morning, and if I leave it too long, there won't be a spot available. Would you mind taking me home after we leave Logan's?" She took a breath. "We can work on the finalization at my house, since it probably won't take too long. I just want you to make sure I haven't forgotten anything."

That was what she was worried about? That was an easy one. "That's fine. It'll even play into our reason for needing to leave early. You're in Brooklyn, right?"

Sam knew that the street sweepers were a big thing in a lot of the neighborhoods with cars needing to be moved in anticipation of them coming. They were programmed for different days, and it was always a hassle for everyone— the city workers included.

"Yes. Thank you. I really appreciate it."

"If you want you can just send me the presentation, if you don't feel like working that late."

"I'd rather you look it over before I send it to you, since you don't know how to work the program. That way it's done and dusted, and you can just forward it to Todd."

"Are you sure?"

"I am. You'll be doing me a favor anyway because I won't need to catch the train back to Brooklyn tonight."

"As if it'll be any faster to drive." He sent her a smile to let her know that he was kidding, although not about the traffic. "You're doing me an even bigger favor in coming to dinner. Are you sure you don't want to back out?"

"I'm sure. How about you?"

"Hell, I never wanted to go in the first place. But I love my brother, so I'll see it through." He held up a bottle that sat between their seats. "I did bring wine, though. I figured we all might need it."

Lucy bit her lip.

"What?" he asked.

"Harper probably can't drink any of it. With the pregnancy and all."

"Damn. Of course she can't."

"It's not a big deal. They might want to serve it to your parents, or they can save it for a later date."

He shook his head. "I think maybe we'll just have a glass at your house while we're working on the presentation. Unless you don't drink either."

"Oh, I drink, all right." She laughed. "Okay, so that came out a little too enthusiastic, so let me try again. I only drink in moderation."

"Such a sensible answer. But since I'm driving, I'm the one who'll be watching what I drink."

They pulled up to Logan and Harper's place right at seven. Which was good because they wouldn't need to sit around trying to think of small talk, since his parents would undoubtedly already be there. They were always fashionably early to everything. Not too early, though. No one wanted to seem too eager.

He found a spot to park and glanced over at Lucy. "It's not too late to back out."

"Yes, it is. Even if it weren't, though, we'd still

go in. This will be good, Sam. Hopefully it'll be a new start for you and your dad."

"Always the optimist. It's what I like about you." He squeezed her hand, more for his own sake than hers. "Let's go."

Lucy was not at all nervous, surprisingly, as Harper opened the door and greeted them. "So glad you guys could come." She chuckled. "And I mean *really* glad."

"They're already here?"

"Yep. Arrived about a half hour ago. We've sat around mainly sizing each other up and trying to find small talk topics that haven't already been covered. I didn't think this would be so hard. Although Logan has been wonderful. He hasn't left my side. Well, at least until the doorbell rang."

She ushered them inside.

"Congratulations again, by the way," Lucy whispered.

Harper took her hand and gave it a squeeze, much like Sam had done a few minutes ago. "Thanks. Wish us luck when we share the news."

"Consider it wished."

Sam hadn't said anything so far, but when she glanced up at him she saw that his jaw was so tight it looked ready to break.

She pressed her arm to his. "It's going to be

okay, Sam. It's only one point in time. Just remember that. No matter how uncomfortable things might get, it's only a small blip in a lifetime of experiences."

He visibly relaxed. "Thanks, Luce. I needed to hear that."

They went into the room. The woman who'd come by Sam's office a month ago stood and came over to them, kissing Sam on the cheek and then giving her a perfunctory hug. "Nice to see you again."

The embrace might have been stiff, but her words were not as chilly as they'd been the last time they'd met. Or maybe it was Lucy's imagination. Sam had pegged her right when he'd said she was an optimist. She always tried to see the best in people. And although Matt had sent her into a tailspin and made everything dark and hopeless looking, her sister had been the one to give her the advice about this only being one point in time and that it wasn't forever. That had meant so much to her that she'd felt she needed to tell Sam the same thing.

It seemed to work.

Biddie went back over to sit with her husband, and Lucy whispered up to Sam, "Consider this nudge number one. Take me over there and introduce me to him."

He took a visible breath before heading toward the man who was sitting on the sofa, his back ramrod straight, although he was thinner than Lucy had somehow pictured him. But the aura he gave off was one of power. She imagined he cowed a whole lot of people. But Lucy wasn't one of them. Ah... Sam wasn't either, which was why they'd probably butted heads over the years. The realization came to her in a flash.

Sam stopped in front of his father, who didn't stand to greet them. Lucy instinctively lifted her chin and prepared for battle. Then belatedly, the man did actually rise from his seat. "How was Uruguay? I didn't get a chance to ask you at the fundraiser."

"It was fine, Dad." He nodded toward her. "This is a coworker from the hospital, Lucy Galeano. We're working on the planning for a new department. Lucy, this is my dad, Carter Grant."

Carter held out his hand, and his grip was firm but not a death squeeze, which she'd been halfway expecting.

"Nice to meet you," she murmured. "I met your wife a few weeks ago at the hospital."

Logan appeared from the kitchen and came over. "Dinner is ready. Everything is in the kitchen, we're doing this buffet style—as in everyone will serve themselves."

If Biddie or Carter seemed surprised by that, they hid it well. And suddenly she realized that was how they were. Even if they hated something, she doubted anyone would realize it. At least not right away. Those cuts would, instead, come in a million subtle ways. And that had to have made it hard on their kids. Carter had made no effort to shake Sam's hand or fold him into an embrace the way her own father would have done if he'd had a son. That didn't make him necessarily a bad man but maybe one who felt a need to protect himself.

Sam did that too, even though he probably didn't realize it.

They followed Logan and Harper into a large kitchen area. "It smells wonderful in here," Lucy said.

Harper came over and looped her arm through hers. "I knew I was going to like you. I'm just now starting to like the smell of food again." Her voice was soft—only meant for Lucy. "The last time I saw Sam, he told me how much you were helping with the new program."

Lucy smiled. "I really haven't done all that much. But we are trying to get a presentation ready for tomorrow. So I'm sorry we have to run out on you early."

She slid that in, lifting the level of her voice

enough for Biddie and Carter to hopefully hear the apology.

Harper nodded. "Sam told us. We do appreciate you coming anyway, though."

Then she went to the head of what looked to be a long line of food to join Logan.

He named the dishes and motioned to the plates and cutlery near the front. He then smiled. "There are no assigned seats at the table, so sit anywhere you want."

Lucy heard Sam chuckle under his breath, and she glanced over and whispered, "I take it that's not the way things were done when you were kids."

"Nope. But I'm glad Logan is setting the standard, and I know him well enough to know he'll stick to it, whether Dad likes it or not."

"Mom and Dad, why don't you go first." Logan came back and led the pair to the front of the line. And there was no way you would have known that Biddie and Carter hadn't done this a million times before. Although they probably had, since they undoubtedly attended a lot of charitable functions, some of them probably serving buffet dinners much like this one.

They made it through the line, and then Harper motioned for her and Sam to go ahead.

As Lucy picked up her plate, she murmured to her, "Is there anything I can do to help?"

Harper smiled. "Just be you. That's what will help."

That surprised her. Lucy knew of Harper, but she didn't really *know* her. And since the couple both worked with neonates, they didn't really deal with the population segment that frequented Lucy's cubicle over in PT. But hospitals were huge gossip mills, so maybe they'd heard things about her. Hopefully good things.

Once everyone had their plates, they started eating. Carter turned to Sam and said, "Tell me about this new venture you're heading at the hospital."

As soon as she heard the words, Lucy knew they would set the wrong tone with Sam. He would not see this as a venture but as a mission. She used her knee to nudge him under the table. One side of his mouth went up, saying he'd felt the slight pressure and it had struck him as humorous.

"We're hoping to help people who are unable to show emotion."

¡Dios! Lucy had just taken a drink of water and it went down the wrong pipe, and she started coughing into her elbow. Loudly. When she glanced at Harper, horrified and trying to stop

the spasms before they came to the surface, she found that the other woman was dabbing her mouth with a napkin, trying to hide her own smile.

Had Sam said that on purpose?

Lucy gained control of herself and added, "It's kind of a fascinating field. It's for people who've had something affect some of the nerves of their face, leaving those muscles paralyzed. Some are unable to smile or even move their eyes. Sam will be heading a department that will transplant muscles and nerves that will help change that."

Biddie smiled, maybe trying to show that her own muscles weren't actually impaired. "That does sound fascinating. I never knew such a thing existed."

Sam seemed to catch on to what he should be doing and expanded on the field, trying to use terms that laymen could understand. "We're hoping it will be up and running a few months from now."

"Are you looking for grant money?" Carter asked the question, and no one said anything for several long seconds. Sam had hinted that Carter probably wouldn't want to fund a program that he was involved with. But Lucy wasn't getting that vibe. Still, she was pretty sure that Sam would be leery of any money that came from Carter's own coffers.

"We've already gotten quite a bit of funding with more being pledged daily."

Parry and feint. A decent strategy on Sam's part. He wasn't saying that they couldn't use the funding while at the same time making sure that Carter knew he hadn't come here to ask for money.

The man nodded. "I saw the press release. I always thought Todd Wells was the right man to lead Manhattan Memorial."

Lucy was pretty sure that was a roundabout way of paying the hospital a compliment for being forward thinking. She crossed her fingers under the table.

"I love the pediatric oncology department. Those kids are the sweetest." Biddie seemed to follow Carter's lead. And the woman probably really did love those kids, since Sam said she went once a week to do a book reading for them. She could always find other charities that had fewer heartbreaking stories. For her to keep going week after week was a testament to an inner strength that Lucy wondered if her son saw.

They talked for a few more minutes about the new department as everyone finished their meal, and then Logan got up and brought in dessert. "I know how much Mom likes flan, so we made this especially for her."

"Oh!" Biddie's smile seemed to widen. "I do love it. Thank you."

Logan served wedges of the dessert onto small plates and served Harper last, bending down to kiss her on the mouth. Then he looked at the group. "Before we start eating, and because I know that Sam and Lucy have to leave soon to finish a project, I have some news to share with all of you." He motioned Harper to stand with him. She did, looping her arms around his waist and gazing up at him. He glanced down at her. "Actually, I'm going to let Harper tell you."

"Okay." Harper lifted up her dessert plate and untaped something from beneath it. When she unfolded it and held it up for everyone to see, there was another period of silence at the table as everyone looked at the unmistakable image on the sheet of paper.

"Do you mean..." Biddie's tentative voice faded away, and her hand went to her mouth.

Harper nodded. "Logan and I are expecting a baby."

"I'm going to be a grandmother?"

"You are."

Biddie threw her napkin onto the table and

got up from her spot, coming around to hug Harper, squeezing tight. When Lucy glanced over at Logan, she saw his mouth was open as if he couldn't quite believe what he was seeing.

Evidently this hadn't been a normal mode of expressing joy in their household. Harper glanced over at Logan, then her arms went around the older woman, a sheen of what looked like tears in her eyes. Lucy had heard that babies could be a source of healing, and she believed it. When she'd seen Sam cradling the infant he'd operated on a few weeks ago, it had done something to Lucy's insides. It had basically turned them to mush.

Not wanting to let on that she and Sam already knew the news, Lucy got up and went over to hug first Logan and then Harper. Sam followed suit, and there were a lot of words of congratulations. The only one who hadn't said anything was Carter, and when she glanced at him, he seemed perfectly stoic, sitting all alone like a statue that was cemented in place.

Then the man with whom Sam had had such conflict over the years suddenly looked over at his wife and his eyes rolled back in his head before falling sideways out of his chair, landing on the floor with a loud thud.

* * *

Sam was the first to his father's side, taking his pulse. Lucy came over with her phone turned to the flashlight function, and he had her flick it back and forth across the man's pupils as Sam pushed his lids open.

"Pulse is good, if just a little bit fast, and pupils are equal and reactive. I think we should call a squad because of his cardiac history, but I think... I think maybe he just fainted."

"Fainted? Carter has never fainted in his life." Biddie's voice shook.

"I know. Logan is already calling the squad. He'll get great care."

Two hours later, dessert forgotten, everyone—including Sarah, who'd rushed over from her office at the family firm—was gathered in a waiting area at the hospital, hoping for some news. Greg Asbury happened to be there late winding up some paperwork and came down to examine him. He appeared in the doorway, and the family all stood up. Biddie was twisting her fingers and kept pressing tissues to her eyes although she'd never actually sobbed out loud. Still, Sam sensed she was worried in a way he'd never known her to be.

Greg slid into a chair and waited for everyone to sit back down. Hell, had his dad died? He remembered Lucy's words about no one knowing how much time anyone had left and that he should work on clearing the air.

Had he actually succeeded in doing that at all?

Logan finally broke the silence. "How is he?"

The neurosurgeon actually smiled. "You mean besides being angry as hell about us poking and prodding him? Not that you can tell much of anything from his stony silence."

Sarah actually laughed. "Sounds like Dad."

Yes, it did. Sam had no doubt death would only take his dad by dragging him bodily into the other realm.

"Seriously, though. As far as I can tell he's fine. His MRI came back clean, as did his other tests. The stents are holding. And his gray matter looks good. No signs of a transient ischemic attack."

"So what happened to him?" Sarah asked.

"I think Sam was right—he simply fainted when you told him the news." Greg smiled again. "Congratulations again, by the way. I'd like to keep him overnight for observation, but I doubt very much that he'll let us, so if you'll agree to keep an eye on him and call us at the first sign of trouble, I'll get his discharge papers started."

"Thank God." The words were soft but unmistakable. His mom continued. "I'll take him home. Between me and our housekeeper, we'll keep watch over him tonight."

"I'll spend the night too, if that's okay, Mom." Sarah went over and put an arm around her mother's shoulders, giving her a gentle squeeze. "I'll let everyone know how he is in the morning."

Greg slapped his palms on his knees and stood. "That sounds like a good plan to me. We'll have him out as soon as we can. Be ready for some general grumpiness."

"Truer words were never spoken," said Logan, hugging Harper. "Are you okay?"

"Yes. I'm just glad he's okay. And you know what? I think everything else will be as well."

Logan glanced over at them. "Damn, you two needed to leave, didn't you?"

"It's okay." Lucy sat in a chair, where she'd been ever since they arrived at the hospital. She hadn't said much, but this had to be awkward for her. She hadn't signed up for being roped into a family emergency.

Sam stood. It was after ten. Again. He seemed to be making a habit of getting her home late. "Let's get you back to Brooklyn. We can work on the project tomorrow. I know you've got to move your car."

When all eyes turned to her, Lucy gave a half grin. "Street-sweeper day tomorrow."

There were a couple of groans, saying people knew exactly what she was talking about. "How hard is it going to be for you to find a parking place?" Harper asked.

She shrugged. "It'll be okay."

Or maybe it wouldn't. He thought of something but decided to wait until they got in the car to share it with her.

A few minutes later they were on their way.

"How about if we get your car and bring it back to my place?"

Shock rolled through Lucy's system. "What?" She had to have misunderstood his words.

"Just hear me out. It's going to be almost impossible for you to park at this time of night. By the time we get there it'll be almost eleven. I have two bedrooms. We can pick up some of your things, and you can follow me back."

"I can't put you out like that." But even as she said it, she had to admit it sounded better than circling the block for hours or having to double park, which was always an iffy prospect. This was what she got for having a place that only had street parking. And her parents didn't have any extra spots in front of theirs, since Bella shared the space with them and had a car of her own.

"You won't be putting me out. Besides, I was the one who asked you to come tonight. It's the least I can do."

It sounded harmless enough, and she was pretty exhausted. "You have an extra parking space?"

"My apartment is assigned two spots, so yes. It'll be fine. The place came furnished, so there's actually a bed in the second bedroom, which I couldn't promise if I'd had to furnish it."

"Okay. But only if you're sure."

"I am. If you don't have to be at work right away, we can get up in the morning and go over the presentation and send it off to Todd. No one will ever know that you spent the night. Not even my family."

Relief washed over her. She really hadn't wanted his family to get the wrong idea, and telling them that she was spending the night was sure to send a couple of stray thoughts winging through their synapses. It was human nature.

"Thanks. And I'm so glad your dad is going to be okay."

"Me too." He glanced over as they made their way to Brooklyn. "Thank you for everything tonight. For the advice and for coming with me."

"Not a problem."

The next half hour was spent in silence, and when they pulled up in front of her house, she noted that hers was one of the only vehicles still on this side of the road. Most people had been smart enough to move theirs hours ago. "That'll teach me not to leave a spare key with my family. I'll just be a minute."

She ran in and gathered a few necessities and her computer, putting an extra flash drive in the bag she carried the device in. Then she ran back out the door and got into her car, texting her mom really quick and letting her know she'd be spending the night in Manhattan with a friend. Otherwise she would worry.

I'll send another text when I get there.

Her mom sent a text back.

Okay. Have fun.

She didn't even ask if it was a male friend or a female friend. Maybe because she'd been so devastated over the breakup with Matt that she would have never guessed that Lucy had actually kissed another man.

And liked it.

She then texted Sam.

I'm ready whenever you are.

He answered by flicking his brights on and off and then pulled into the street, waiting until she was behind him before setting off and heading back to Manhattan.

CHAPTER EIGHT

IT WAS AFTER midnight when they finally arrived back at his apartment complex. He'd texted Lucy his address before they left in case he lost her, but she'd stuck to him like glue, pulling several almost crazy moves to keep up with him. He eased his vehicle into the 2101 A parking place and waited for her to take the 2101 B spot. He'd never actually thought he'd need the second one, but he'd wanted an extra bedroom just in case he had a guest or wanted to convert it into an office or workout space. But the truth was he wasn't actually here enough to do that, pretty much just coming home to sleep and going back to work the next day.

And as for having company? He never had. He wasn't even sure if the bed had sheets on it, although the apartment had come with several sets of linens.

He got out of the car and waited for Lucy, taking her two bags, one a gym bag that probably held a change of clothes and the other a computer case. "I have a laptop, you know."

"I figured, but I know mine's quirks and the PowerPoint version that I like the best is on it." She yawned. "I have to admit I was having trouble staying awake the last several miles."

"I'm sorry. I should have thought to send you home on a train rather than dragging you with me to the hospital."

"No. I wanted to be there. I'm just so glad he's okay. It was worth a little loss of sleep."

"I can't believe he fainted. I've never known my dad to show any weakness outside of his infarction a few years back. Even then, Logan had a hell of a time trying to convince him that he needed to get stents."

"I'm sure he's mad that he did. That's probably what Greg was seeing. Anger at himself rather than at anyone at the hospital. And that was a pretty big piece of news. If he was trying to contain his emotions by holding his breath, it could have slowed his heart rate enough to send him into bradycardia. Kind of like a child who holds his breath, then faints and then starts breathing normally again."

"Greg knows my dad pretty well and pulled me aside after talking to the family. That was his hunch as well—that temporary bradycardia caused him to faint."

"I can't help but think your parents are ecstatic about the baby. Hopefully it will soften your dad's heart a little bit. Raising kids is stressful and not everyone gets it right all the time. But grandkids? From what I've heard, that's when people have the most fun because they can enjoy those little ones without the strain of discipline and all of the things that go with parenting."

"Not disciplining? That sounds like torture for my dad." But he laughed as he said it.

They reached his apartment, and he used a keypad to let himself in. His place wasn't super fancy, but it did what he needed it to do. Sam had never had a need for the things that wealth brought. He lived for his work. It was where he was the happiest. Priscilla would probably never understand that. And since living the way the other preferred to would only lead to a life of misery for one or both of them, he'd broken things off. The cursing she'd done in Spanish when he had hadn't been nearly as cute as Lucy's had been that day in the conference room. But then again, it hadn't been aimed at him either. She would be fine. From what it looked like, her modeling career would soon eclipse her career in medicine. And it would bring her everything she wanted out of life.

Lucy, on the other hand, seemed to love what she did for a living. And from her comments about the contract, she wasn't worried about the money aspect of it any more than he was.

And that was something he didn't want to look too closely at.

She was right about being tired. He was feeling the effects of the long day and the stress of spending time with his parents. Anything he might've been thinking right now was the result of that. So he needed to save things that needed methodical and rational consideration for morning.

"I think you're probably right about the grandkids. But as for softening my dad? I guess time will tell. He'll have to learn a whole new way of dealing with people and kids for it to work, though. After everything Logan and Harper have been through, I know my brother isn't going to take any crap from him this time around. And I don't blame him."

"And are you going to take any crap from him?"

"I think I got most of that out of my system when I was fifteen." He took her stuff to the second bedroom and set it on the bed. "I sure hope there are sheets on this thing."

Lucy pulled the covers away from the pillows and revealed pillowcases and sheets that looked clean and crisp. "They probably changed these right before you moved in."

"If you say so." He glanced at a closet in the hallway. "Looks like there are some spares in here if you want me to change them out."

"It's fine. It's not like you've lived here that long." She glanced at him before sitting on the edge of the bed. "You were saying something about getting it out of your system when you were fifteen?"

He shook his head. "It doesn't matter." The last thing she needed to hear when she was tired was the stupid stuff he'd done when he was younger.

"No, really. I want to know what you did. Go to wild parties? Get someone pregnant?"

What would have happened if Priscilla had wound up pregnant when they were together? Not something he wanted to even contemplate.

"Nothing like that." He paused. "I actually got arrested while at a protest march."

"Arrested. Seriously? When you were fifteen?" She actually looked shocked. "What kind of march was it?"

He made a clicking sound with his tongue. "Yeah…it was about real weighty stuff."

Her eyes widened. "World peace? Wars? Politics?"

"Homework."

There wasn't a sound for about fifteen seconds, and then she started laughing. The sound started low and grew until she was gasping for breath. He was afraid for a second that she might pass out herself. He sat down beside her.

"You're lying." Her breathing was still ragged.

He held up a hand, three fingers raised. "I swear. A bunch of schools participated, skipping class and going to a park—Pirius Park, actually—to protest the homework load we were getting. Of course, several schools being there meant that rival football teams eventually met up and some fights ensued, and well…the police showed up and handcuffed anyone they could catch. Me included. My dad was not happy. At all. But you know what? He never raised his voice to me and only grounded me for a week. But he did turn the screws and try to guilt me into coming to work for his company."

"Okay, wow. You've got me beat on the teenage rebellion. I never got arrested. Mine was much milder, and I was seventeen at the time."

This he had to hear. "What did you do, Lucy?"

"I got this." She twisted on the bed and pulled the top of her tank top aside and revealed ink.

His brows went up, and he leaned in to get a closer look. It was a black line tattoo on her left shoulder. About an inch and a half square, it was the image of a tiny bunny sitting up on its haunches holding a piece of clover. His finger touched it. "Cute. Was there an occasion?"

"I got it for my sister." She shrugged the shoulder. "I'm not even sure why. She never asked me to. But there was just this sense of need inside of me when I saw it in the window of a tattoo parlor. I couldn't resist. And I love it. I don't regret getting it done."

"I like your rebellion a hell of a lot better than mine." He could definitely relate to the sense of need that couldn't be resisted. "Did you get in trouble?"

"No. My dad is against tattoos, but he never said anything. And my mom said she liked it. But not to do it again." Lucy laughed and looked up at him, her eyes soft and dreamy. "Have you ever done anything you liked but shouldn't do again?"

He swallowed before answering. "I have. Not too long ago, actually."

"Mmm… Yeah. Me too."

His eyes swept over her tattoo again. She

might have been telling the truth about her reasons for getting it, but when he looked at the tattoo, he saw her in the figure. The bunny was cute and perky and full of vibrant hope. Just like Lucy. He envied her for being able to be like that. Sam had always felt like he had a dark undercurrent that never quite went away no matter what he did.

"I like this." His fingers brushed across it again. "It fits you."

Before he could stop himself he leaned over and kissed it. He'd meant to touch it and leave, but her skin was soft and clean, and the scent coming off of her was like the freshest of meadows. Just like the place the bunny in her tattoo might inhabit.

Her head tilted forward and she moved her long hair to the side as if opening the site up for his exploration. But he didn't dare. Because if he did, he might not stop.

"Luce." The word was muttered an inch away from her skin, helpless to move, as if he were tethered there by an unseen string.

She lifted her hand, her palm cradling the back of his head. "I like *that*."

There was no question about what she meant. "Are you sure?"

She gave a husky laugh. "It isn't just teenagers who rebel. Sometimes adults need to visit dangerous places too."

Nerve endings all across his body prickled to life.

"Is this a dangerous place?" He kissed the tattoo again.

"Not even warm."

God, her voice. How could a simple change in tone drive him crazy? But it did.

"How about here?" He kissed the nape of her neck, letting his lips trail to a shadowed spot behind her ear.

"Warmer. So, so warm."

He bit the edge of her ear, nibbling his way to the lobe, taking it and the small glittering diamond that sat on it into his mouth.

"Ahh…" The sound was thick, and he recognized the need in it because he was feeling it too.

"Warmer?"

"Much."

He moved to the edge of her mouth and kissed the corner of it. "And here. Is this warmer?"

"No, Sam, that is hot. And I want it now." She turned her head, and this time it was her kissing him with a fervor that drove his body into high gear, and they'd barely even begun to explore each other. But they would. He just had to hold on long enough to get the job done.

Job? Oh, hell no. This wasn't work. This was pure unadulterated pleasure.

Or maybe it was adulterated. No. Wrong word. He was looking for the word *adultery*. No, that was wrong too. Neither of them was married. Neither of them had any entanglements. They were both free to do whatever they wanted. For however long they desired.

And damn if Sam didn't want to do it for a long, long time.

He pressed her back onto the mattress and pulled the stretchy material of her top away from her shoulder, pressing his mouth to the side of her neck and applying gentle suction. What was a little rebellion? He needed it.

As if answering him, she arched her back and pressed into his mouth. "Yes!"

Sam sucked harder, and she gasped, hands coming up and holding him against her neck, sending a tremendous need over him.

He rose up and grabbed his shirt, going to haul it over his head, only to realize it was buttoned and not his normal polo shirt. "Damn!"

Her eyes opened, and she looked at what he was doing before pushing his hands away. "Let me." She sat up, his thighs straddling her hips, and reached up, undoing his buttons one at a time.

He touched her neck, realizing the redness there was caused by him. "I left a mark."

"Yes. You did." Her smile was the sexiest thing he had ever seen.

Then her hands were pushing the shirt down his arms and helping him shrug out of it. She might not care about the mark now, but she would when they eventually had to leave this room. But he could worry about that later.

Any hint of tiredness had vanished, and in its place was a need he'd never felt before. Lucy was gorgeous and sexy and everything that was good in a person, and for tonight, she was his.

And if you want more than tonight?

He swiped the thought away, admonishing himself to stay in the here and now.

Here and now was exactly where he wanted to be. Here with this woman and now, in this moment.

It was good enough. It would have to be because he couldn't ask for any more than that.

Her fingers traced over his pecs and across his nipples, sending a shudder over him. But she didn't pause, just went down his sides, her short nails adding an extra layer of texture to the already heady sensation. She hit a ticklish spot on his ribs and his skin rippled, but he'd never felt less like laughing than he did right now because the tickle was mixed with a sensuality that swept everything else to the side.

His hands went to her sides and gripped her, even though he was pretty sure she wasn't going to slip away into the night, but he needed to touch her—to hold her—to make himself believe that she was really here with him.

He took hold of the bottom of her white tank top, marveling in the contrast between it and the deep tan of her skin, and slid it up, missing the feel of her hands on his skin as she helped him get the garment over her head. He tossed it to where his crumpled shirt lay on the floor.

Her nude bra, lacy enough to show glimpses of her breasts, drew his hands, and he curved his palms over the soft flesh. Lucy's nipples were tight and pushed into his flesh, and the need to get her bra off came fast and hard. He undid the hooks in back and then flung the undergarment away.

This woman had everything a man could want, and he took a moment to gaze at her before smoothing her hair back from her face and looking into her eyes. "You are so beautiful. Do you know that?"

She smiled. "So are you. You're a walking advertisement for plastic surgery."

That scraped across a raw spot no one could

see. His dad had ridiculed him for going into his field.

Lucy sat up straighter and peered at him. "What?"

"Nothing."

She cupped his face. "Hey. I didn't mean that in a bad way. You're just gorgeous. And I can't think of a way to say it that will adequately get that across."

He relaxed. "Same here." He leaned over and kissed her forehead and then pressed his brow against it. Why was he picking apart her words rather than making love to her?

He didn't know, but that stopped now. He stood, and then as she watched, he undid his jeans and slid out of them, taking his briefs down with them. Then his shoes and socks followed.

"Wow." She blinked, but her eyes were not on his face but on his…

That made him laugh. "Want to play footsie with me again?"

She licked her lips. "I just might. But I wouldn't be using my foot."

His flesh jerked and she moved closer, but he shook his head. "Not this time." Then he scooped her off the bed and pivoted so that the back of his knees were against the mattress. He lowered himself onto it. "I have other ideas."

Sam settled her onto him so that she was doing what he'd done earlier, straddling his thighs. He bunched her skirt and settled her on him so that his erection was tight against her. It was heaven on earth. "Can you reach my nightstand drawer?"

Her head twisted to look. "I think so." She leaned over, needing to go back up on her knees to get to the pull. She slid it open and reached inside. "Looking for these?"

"Yes." He held his hand out for the unopened box of condoms, but she shook her head.

"I don't think you've earned the right to these yet."

He laughed. "Earned the right?"

"You heard me." She set the box on the bed and then, still up on her knees, she came back in front of him and looked down at him, her fingers tracing his temples, his nose and then trailing down to his mouth.

Her breasts were right in front of him, and he realized what she wanted. And he was more than happy to oblige. Splaying his hands on her back, he used gentle pressure to move her forward, kissing between the soft mounds and working his way over the top of the first one, without ever touching her nipple. When he started to do the same with her other breast, she made a sound.

"What?" he said. "I'm earning my keep."

Her fingers buried themselves in his hair. "You're really not."

"Then show me." His brows went up in challenge.

She drew his head to her body in a way that left no doubt as to what she wanted. Finally. He took her nipple in his mouth and used his tongue to slide over the tight skin before suckling it, holding her in place with light pressure from his teeth.

"*Dios. ¡Sí! ¡Así!*"

The Spanish words telling him to do it "just like that" crashed into him like a wave—big and powerful and stripping any willpower he had left.

He reached for the box and made quick work out of opening it and sheathing himself. When she went to climb off of him as if to finish undressing, he grabbed her hips. "No. Just come here."

She settled back on top of him while he kissed her neck, her chin, her eyes and finally took her mouth, his tongue thrusting deep and mimicking what his body was about to do. His arm went around her hips and jerked them forward until he was gripped between his stomach and hers, reveling in the pressure and knowing better things were soon to come. He kept kissing her, even as his hands on her hips guided her up until he found the elastic of her panties and slid them aside, finding a moist heat that drove his mind into a frenzy of want and need. Pulling her back to him, he drew her down, found her in a single attempt and thrust upward, even as he settled her fully onto him.

He closed his eyes and absorbed the sensation, not daring to move, and holding her in place so she didn't either.

"Damn. It's so good. So, so good." His muttered words against her mouth were all he could manage as they poised precariously on the edge of a cliff. A cliff of firsts that, once fallen off of, could never be revisited. He never wanted to forget this moment.

"Yes, it is." Her mouth reached for his. "But I want more, Sam. I *need* more."

The words tickled at a place in his subconscious, but he ignored it, knowing she hadn't meant her words that way.

He gave her what she wanted, easing his grip on her hips and helping her move on him. The ripples of pleasure were indescribable as her body slid up and away from him before returning time and time again as if sating a deep need.

Each pump brought a greater craving that he soon would be powerless to resist.

Up and down. Engulfing him fully and then up until only the tip had contact. God. It was the portals of heaven coming down to where he was.

Lucy's arms wrapped around his neck and head as she rose and fell, her tempo increasing, raising the level of his insanity. She muttered words in Spanish that he no longer tried to translate. He was powerless to. Powerless to do anything else but hang on and let her do what she wanted, to let her get what she needed from him and to give it back in spades.

The rhythm changed, becoming one of utter desperation, until she gave a long keening cry, her head thrown back as she continued to rise and fall in quick staccato movements of her hips. And in an instant, he was gone, tumbling over that cliff he'd imagined earlier and falling all the way to the bottom. The crash on impact, when it came, overwhelmed him and brought a coarse shout that he couldn't have contained if he'd tried.

Sam couldn't think, couldn't breathe, couldn't move as Lucy slowed her pace, the fingers that had gripped his shoulders easing and becoming soothing touches that helped him transition from tornado-like furor to a calm sea that cradled and comforted. His arms went around her and held her against him as all movements stopped.

He didn't want to get up. Didn't want this moment to end, because when it did...

No. He didn't want to think beyond the feel of her skin against his.

"Sam?" Her low voice pulled him from whatever dreamland he'd been in, and he took a deep breath, hoping she wasn't going to say anything profound or weighty. Or talk about needing more from him. He didn't think he could handle it right now.

"Yep?" It took everything in him to get that one word out. And he braced himself for whatever she was about to say.

She leaned back and looked at him. "I think you earned it."

His mind scrambled, trying to figure out what she was talking about, then her fingers walked across the mattress until she reached the box that was still beside her hip. She tapped it, and her eyebrows gave a sexy wiggle.

All of a sudden he laughed and laid back, dragging her with him. He shut his eyes. It was going to be okay. Everything would be okay.

CHAPTER NINE

LUCY WOKE UP feeling a little stiff and out of sorts. And very, very tired. Where was she?

She glanced to the side and saw an end table, the drawer still halfway open. Oh, God. They really had...

She sat up in an instant and listened, trying to figure out where Sam was. He wasn't in the room or in the adjoining bathroom, since that door was open and the lights were out.

How many times had they made love last night?

Too many. She should've been stretching her arms up and relishing what had happened. But in the way that it always was with her, her emotions were cramped and small and hiding in a corner because they knew she was not going to be happy to see them.

Why? It was just sex. Great, uninhibited sex like she'd never had before in her life.

Still listening for Sam, her mind crouched,

looking at the bundle of feelings that were shrinking away as if trying very hard to protect her from the truth. Again, why? People had sex all the time. It was no big deal. It wasn't like it was her first time. And she'd wanted this to happen almost from the moment she laid eyes on him. All of that had happened in less than a month.

Remember Matt? Things happened fast with him too. So, so fast.

She frowned, a sliver of anger coming over her. Sam wasn't Matt. And they weren't committed. Or engaged.

But it's what you're hoping for. All in under a month. Just like with Matt.

"It's not the same!" Her words were low, and she glanced at the door to make sure Sam wasn't standing there listening. He wasn't.

Her thoughts strayed again to that dark corner, and slowly her feelings crept out into the open where she could see them. *Oh, God, no.* She closed her eyes as a truth—a truth that was every bit as catastrophic to her senses as last night had been—revealed itself.

She'd done the unthinkable. Done exactly what she'd warned herself over and over not to do.

She'd fallen in love with Sam.

And it hadn't happened last night either. It had been there for the past couple of weeks—she just hadn't recognized it. Which made it even worse.

What had he told her? That he didn't want to be involved with anyone. That he probably would *never* want to be involved with anyone ever again. He'd never lied to her or promised her anything. They'd wanted each other and had acted on it. It wasn't his fault. And it really wasn't hers either. As long as she didn't press him to give her something more than he already had.

He couldn't know. She was going to have to work very hard to not let him see what had happened. The bunny on her shoulder burned with a fire that seared her conscience. She was horrible at hiding her feelings. The worst.

Maybe it was why Matt had left her a note instead of facing her.

Well, she was going to have to learn quick or ruin everything she'd worked so hard for. She doubted he'd throw her off the team, but she might not be able to stay on it if she couldn't keep her feelings in check. If she couldn't make him believe that last night would never happen again, that it had meant nothing.

It was a lie. It had meant everything. But no matter how she looked at it, she couldn't see a way in which this would work out, unless he'd fallen in love with her too.

And that seemed improbable if not impossible, given everything he'd told her.

Where was he? Maybe he was cooking a gourmet breakfast for her, waiting to tell her how much last night meant to him.

Lucy wrinkled her nose as if sniffing the air. Nothing. And there wasn't a sound coming from anywhere. No sounds of toilets flushing or water running or of bare feet walking across the hardwood floors of his little apartment.

Gingerly she got out of bed and thanked God that she'd brought a change of clothing with her. Her clothes were still on the floor, but Sam's were not. He'd evidently picked them up. She swallowed. The box of condoms was gone as well, and she didn't see it in the drawer of the side table either. She pushed the drawer shut and caught sight of something else. It wasn't the missing box.

A sense of horror came over her. There was a slip of paper on one of the pillows at the head of the bed. The pillows that neither one of them had used last night.

She slowly walked over to it, her feet feeling as if they were encased in blocks of concrete, getting heavier with every step. The note was folded, and she wasn't going to be able to read it without touching it. And she didn't want to touch it. She knew exactly what that paper would feel like against her skin.

It would feel like heartbreak. All over again.

She forced her hand to move forward and pick it up, fingers opening the folded portion of it.

Emergency at MMH. Talk later.

He hadn't even signed the note, and she couldn't remember hearing the sound of a phone going off. Which could mean nothing. His phone could have been on vibrate or on the table in the foyer. Or it could mean that he'd simply been looking for an excuse to get out of his own apartment before she woke up and he had to face her.

And talk later? The last thing Lucy wanted to do was talk. Not until she'd had a chance to stop and think about the ramifications of everything that had happened.

Whichever scenario was the case, thank God she had her own car and didn't have to be at work until later this afternoon. Because she was going to get dressed—she glanced down, realizing she was still completely naked—drive home and figure out a way to get past this. One that didn't involve leaving her job or quitting the team. She wouldn't have to leave her job, since they worked in completely different parts of the hospital and she would rarely have to see him. But leaving the team?

Even the thought of meeting with him and finishing the work on that presentation filled her with a sense of nausea. And the idea of talking things through with him? When his eyes met hers, she had visions of him shrinking away after seeing the truth written all over her face.

No, he wouldn't. Because she was about to become the best damned actress MMH had ever seen. No one would guess. Not Logan, not Harper and definitely not Sam. She'd taken a chance with Matt and had come out on the losing end. She was not about to do that a second time.

Nor was she going to face Sam over the keyboard of a computer and work on that project. She couldn't. Not today.

Yanking on her clothes, she went out to the dining room table, hoping he had just left and wouldn't be home for a while. Then she pulled her computer out of its bag and opened it, sitting in one of his chairs and getting to work.

In a half hour, she'd done everything she needed to do and put the extra flash drive into the slot and loaded her work onto it. Then, retrieving the note from the pillow, she brought it to where her computer sat on the table. She pulled an ink pen from her bag and sat down again, staring at the note for a long time. Then she added a reply onto it.

No need to talk. Project ready for Todd. See copy on flash drive.

She didn't sign her name either, just folded the note back up and dropped the tiny device on top of it. Then she gathered all of her stuff and left the apartment.

Lucy glanced at her phone and saw that she'd missed a call from him. Swallowing, she didn't try to return it. Right now, she just wanted to get out.

When she got to the parking lot, she was grateful to see that the space next her car's was empty. Maybe her feelings were just an overflow of giddiness from what had happened last night. Except the discovery of those emotions had not had the slightest resemblance to anything she'd felt last night. They were somber and sad and knew exactly what would happen once she recognized them.

She threw her stuff into the back seat and drove home as fast as she could. Fortunately the street sweeper had already come and gone and she was able to park fairly close to her little house. But when she got out, her sister was evidently waiting for her and came down the sidewalk toward her. She took Lucy's computer bag without a word, looking into her face and then a little bit lower, her cane leaning against her thigh.

"What happened?"

Dios. She couldn't even hide the truth for five seconds without someone guessing it. How on earth was she going to keep it from Sam?

She dropped her overnight bag onto the sidewalk and covered her face with her hands, silent tears streaming down her face.

"Oh, Luce...tell me. Tell me, please."

"I—I... Oh, God, I fell in love."

Bella evidently guessed that this was not good news because she held her as Lucy sobbed onto her shoulder. "I'm so sorry, honey. So, so sorry. Is there no chance?"

"None." Even as she said it, she knew it was true. Because she wasn't willing to take a chance on being rejected again. She wasn't going to tell Sam. Or her mom or dad. Or anyone else. "You can't say anything, Bell. Promise me."

"I promise. But promise me you won't give up."

"I can't. But what I can promise you is that it's not going to keep me from doing what I love doing."

"Good. You know I'm here for you, right?"

Lucy leaned back and gave her sister a watery

smile. "I do. And thank you for that." She gave a shrug. "At least there are no wedding plans to cancel this time."

With that, Bella walked her up to her front porch and came inside the house. "You may not want it right now, but I'm going to make you some strong coffee. But not before you lie down and get some sleep."

"How did you guess?"

"I just know. But there's also this." She touched a spot on Lucy's neck.

She put a hand up, remembering the second that mark had happened. A shudder went through her. Oh, God!

She hoped she had something to cover that up with.

Bella kissed her cheek. "Now, go get cleaned up. I'll wake you up before you need to go to work."

She would have asked her sister how she knew what time that would be, but she didn't. Because like her sister had said—she knew. Just like she always did.

Sam was exhausted. A half hour after he'd finally fallen asleep last night, he'd gotten a call that a child had fallen off a step and caught her upper lip on a piece of fencing. It had ripped through all the layers, laying the flesh wide open. Anyone in the ER could have sutured it up, but those doctors also knew that getting the lip margins to perfectly meet was tricky business. It could look right now, but later on any deviation in those edges would be visible as the child grew. So they'd called Sam.

He'd only had time to write a quick note to Lucy and drive to the hospital. Once he'd finished the repair, he checked his phone and saw no messages from Lucy, so he tried to call her and got no response. Either she was still asleep, which was understandable, or she was dreading seeing him again.

He wanted to believe that last night was a mistake, but he couldn't quite bring himself to that point. Sex with her had been like nothing he'd ever experienced before. But the fact that he already wanted it again was a wake-up call. He'd told her the truth. He was not good at relationships. Not with his parents, not with Priscilla. Hell, he didn't even get along with his siblings sometimes. He hated having his emotions exposed and examined…even by his own mind.

And yet Lucy was so good. So kind. And so giving, whether in bed or in life.

He swallowed, thinking about what she'd said about her ex. She'd been hurt in the worst possible way by someone she'd loved. Could he risk hurting her if things crashed and burned like they had with Priscilla?

Maybe she didn't even want anything from him. It could be that he was making a crisis out of something that simply wasn't there.

I want more, Sam. I need *more.*

She'd said it in the heat of passion, but even then the words had scraped at something inside of him. Because while he might have been able to give her more in a physical sense, he wasn't sure he had it in him to give her more emotionally.

Plus, he'd gotten a text from Todd asking if they could host the team from New York's Grayson Specialty Hospital sooner than they'd anticipated. They could come next week if Sam could pull the team together for the Q&A. Todd had also asked about the work he and Lucy had done on the protocol. He told the man he'd have it by the end of the day, but the thought of texting Lucy again made his chest hurt. He was going to have to face her sometime, but it was kind of like his dad. Sam's comfort meter was dialed to avoidance right now.

The fact that she hadn't called him back made him think she felt pretty much the same way, that she was in no hurry to try to figure this thing out. Maybe he could just text her and ask her to forward the presentation file to Todd. But he wasn't going to do that right now, not when exhaustion was pulling at every cell of his body.

So he went back to his office and stretched out on the very uncomfortable futon that the last occupant had left in there and did his best to shut off his mind even as he shut his eyes.

Sam kicked back to consciousness, reaching for something that wasn't there and almost falling off the bed in the process. His eyes popped open.

It wasn't a bed, it was a narrow couch, and the thing he'd been reaching for...

Wasn't there. And probably never would be.

Great. He glanced at his watch and saw that it was a little after one. He'd been asleep for almost four hours. He sat up and scrubbed a hand across his face. It was going to be a long day.

Checking his phone and scrolling through several messages, he noted there was still nothing from Lucy. No word on the project or if she'd even driven home. Surely she wasn't waiting at his apartment for him?

No. That didn't sound like something she would do. But what she would do...

He dragged his hands through his hair and decided to head down to the first floor. Catching the elevator and leaning his head against the wall of the empty car, he tried to run over what he was going to say to her. Nothing sounded appropriate for work.

Or really anywhere, since most everything that popped into his head started off with, *I'm sorry.*

He exited into the main lobby of the hospital and took a right, heading down the corridor that led to the PT department, the big sign overhead stating that he was entering the Manhattan Memorial Hospital Physical Therapy and Wellness Center. He paused at the door before pushing through it with a sense of determination. The sooner they cleared the air, the better for both of them.

Then he heard a familiar sound. A quacking sound that came from his left. There sat Lucy as cheerful as ever, as if nothing had happened to change her world. So why was she able to bounce back so quickly while he felt he was being sucked down into a pit of quicksand? The more he struggled against it, the greater the suction. He stood and watched her for a second, as fascinated by what she did as he had been the last time he visited this department. This child wasn't Devon but was instead a little girl who was actually sitting on top of one of those exercise balls. The child had a puppet of her own, and she and Lucy were carrying on a conversation through the pretend animals. On top of her desk was a spotted dog.

Where had he seen that before?

Spot. That was its name. And Devon. Their tethered-cord patient. He must have visited if the dog was there. Or maybe she'd bought one to replace the one she'd given the boy.

Just then she glanced over, catching sight of him. There was a moment's hesitation, then a brilliant smile lit her face. He frowned. What was she so cheerful about?

Wasn't that just who Lucy was? She was the most optimistic, chipper person he'd ever met. He was glad to see that what happened hadn't seemed to squashed that part of her. She held up a finger to tell him to wait.

Somehow the fact that she seemed so unruffled bothered him. He'd sat and stewed and worried for what seemed like hours before he'd fallen asleep. Or maybe she thought what happened wouldn't change their relationship.

That should've been good news. Except her apparent happiness was making him feel even more miserable. As well it should've. He'd known from the beginning that sleeping with her would bring unintended consequences. But had that stopped him?

No. Because he was too stupid to open his eyes and acknowledge that actions *always* had consequences. Like getting arrested when he was fifteen. Only he was a grown man now. And able to think through things before he did them. Or at least he'd thought he could.

He was tempted to just scribble a note and leave it for her at the information desk, but that wasn't going to solve the problem. They needed to at least have a quick conversation and make sure that they were both good to go on from here. Because if they weren't…

Well, he hadn't thought that far ahead. Would she want to quit the team? Even the thought of that made his gut churn. Maybe it would be easier. But was it what he wanted? He was no longer sure of anything.

Lucy stood up and held the ball while the girl did the same, taking the puppet off her hand. Then a woman, who was probably the child's mom, smiled and said something to Lucy and her daughter before taking the girl's hand and leading her toward the entrance. The girl was limping. He couldn't tell if it was from an injury or if there was some other problem, but that was not why he was here.

Lucy motioned him over. Sam took a deep breath and started toward her.

Her eyes sparkled, and she pointed toward the exercise ball. "Want to have a seat?"

There was no sign of anything on her neck. He could have sworn he'd kissed her hard enough to...

Evidently nothing he'd done last night had left a mark. Except on him.

And her perky words just made his sense of irritation grow. "No, thank you."

"Well, if you insist, there's also a chair."

He sat in it, knowing he was being grumpy and probably was going to act like a jerk pretty soon, but he'd been trying to figure out all morning what he was going to say to her when he finally saw her, but it looked like he needn't have worried.

She went on: "I ended up leaving a flash drive of the presentation on your dining room table, but I have another copy here if you need it for Todd right away. I hope everything with your emergency went well."

"It did—thanks." She was totally not bothered by last night?

Sam was finding that hard to believe. So he decided to come right out with it. "About last night..." The words choked to a halt.

"Yes?" She still had that half smile on her face. Was she hoping for an admission of love? No. He didn't see anything like that in her expression.

He tried again. "I think we were both…"

She was still smiling. "Let me stop you right there. I'm not worried about it if you're not. But I think we can both agree that it's something that shouldn't happen again."

Not exactly what he'd been going to say, but the fact that she'd had no problem getting her words out in a way that was so…unflappable was grating.

His eyes narrowed, and he decided to up his bid to match hers. "I agree."

She slipped her duck puppet on. "Do we need to sign a contract agreeing to that? *Quack-quack.*"

He went very still, the flippant tone sending a shard that went straight to his heart. "I'm glad you find all of this so amusing."

As if she realized she'd gone too far, she set the puppet down. "No, it's not amusing. But I'm also not going to lose sleep over it. I knew where we stood before last night happened, so unless you have something you're dying to say, I suggest we forget it. Getting angsty about it isn't going to help either of us, and we still have to work together on the team." Her brows went up. "Unless you have something to say about that matter as well?"

What could he say? Nothing really, although the idea of working beside her had lost all of its attraction because she might agree to signing a hands-off contract—even in jest—but he wasn't so sure that he could stick to those terms. Because even watching her work with that little girl had warmed his chest. He cared about her. He could admit to that. But the alternative was for one of them to step down, and that held no appeal either. Could he avoid working with her as an individual and keep it strictly to things that were happening within the group as a whole?

Maybe.

"Nope, I have nothing to say. I'm glad things are okay between us."

But were they? Sam wasn't so sure. At least on his side.

"Good," she said. Her smile was back in place. "I have another patient coming in a few minutes, so unless there's something else…"

"No. Nothing else." He stood and looked down at her, still searching for any sign of that kissing mark on her neck. "Thanks for the flash drive. If you have an extra one here, could I borrow it? I promised Todd I'd get it to him today, and it looks like the Q&A with the other hospital is going to take place next week."

"Wow, was that you? Or Todd?"

"Neither. Their hospital decided they wanted to do it earlier than scheduled, so we'll have some scrambling to do to get ready."

"Then I'd better let you go so you can start scrambling." She opened the drawer to her desk. "And here's the flash drive. You can have it. I have the presentation saved on my computer as well, so if you need it, I can make more copies."

"This should be good. Thanks, though."

With that he headed back the way he came, feeling no better about things than when he'd entered the room. He should've been glad that he'd gotten off easy, but the whole idea of that made him feel slightly queasy, as if he were coming down with something.

And he couldn't afford to come down with anything. Not when so many things were riding on his shoulders and counting on him to hold them up. For the first time since he'd been back, he missed Uruguay. But he knew better than most that you couldn't always go back and expect things to be the way they'd been before. Not with Uruguay. And probably not with Lucy either. He couldn't undo what had happened between them. So all he could do was try to make things work the best he could and go on from where they currently stood.

As he was making his way across the lobby, he was shocked to see his dad striding through the big double doors. As always, he was a man on a mission. But he really shouldn't even be out. Not after his fainting episode last night.

Sam moved to intercept him, coming up behind his father. "Dad. What are you doing here?"

Carter Grant stopped in his tracks and stood there for a minute before turning to face him. "I'm looking for my son."

A bitter taste washed up his throat, but he clenched his teeth and willed it away. "Logan is probably in his office."

"No. He's not. And I'm not looking for that son."

For a second he didn't understand what his father was saying, and then he blinked. "You came to see me?"

"Is there somewhere we can go that is a little more private?"

"Are you having a problem? I can page Dr. Asbury and get him down here."

He shook his head. "It's not my health. But last night was a wake-up call."

Hell, he hoped his dad didn't want to talk

about making out his will or money because Sam wasn't in the mood.

"Let's go up to my office."

As soon as they got off the elevator and he opened the door to his space, he realized it was a mistake. His sofa was still pulled into a bed and a blanket was haphazardly thrown over it. But he motioned his father into the room and quickly tossed the blanket aside and righted the sofa. "Have a seat."

"I'll stand, if that's okay. I won't take up a lot of your time."

He tried again. "You really should be at home resting."

His dad shook his head. "Logan came by the house this morning to see how I was doing, and I…" He cleared his throat. "And I decided to come see you."

Sam swallowed. His dad hadn't been the one on his mind this morning. A faint sense of guilt washed over him. "Can't this wait until after you've recovered?"

Carter grunted. "If I'm going to have a heart attack, where better to have it than at the hospital?"

How could he argue with that? He couldn't. And the sooner his father had his say, the sooner

Sam could take him home. "Let's sit. Both of us."

This time, his dad lowered himself onto the couch while Sam spun one of the chairs in front of the desk to face him.

"I know Logan thinks your mother and I played a part in the breakup of their marriage, and maybe he's right. I told him I want to do things differently this time, especially since Harper is expecting."

Sam still didn't see what that had to do with him, so he just sat and waited.

"I was hard on you when you were growing up. If I had it to do over again…well, there's no going back, so let's just say, I regret some things. And when you went away to Uruguay, I wasn't sure I'd ever see you again."

And yet his dad had never contacted him. Not once. But maybe that was pride. Sam, more than anyone, could understand about letting pride get in the way of real conversations. Something he wasn't going to think about right now.

He forced a smile. "Well, you won't have to worry about that anymore."

"I'm sorry?"

Realizing his dad might think he was leaving again, he hurried to set him straight. "I'm here to stay. This new program means a lot to me."

"And the woman from last night? Does she play more of a role than you're letting on?"

"Her name is Lucy." If his father thought he was going to break down and make some big confession, he was sorely mistaken. But Sam could at least extend an olive branch. After all, for his dad to say any of this was something of a miracle. And Sam was smart enough to know that he'd also played a part in their rift over the years. "I don't think so. But I promise to try to communicate more."

Lucy's words about time and trying to make things right while he still could rang in his ears. Maybe his father had come to the same conclusion. But whatever it was, he had to see this as a peace offering. Why else would he have come to see him?

"Thank you, son."

There was that word again. He couldn't remember his dad ever actually calling him that. Maybe there was hope. Or at least a slight glimmer of something that resembled hope.

His dad stood. "Well, I won't take any more of your time. Thanks for letting me say my piece." He held out his hand, and Sam took it and gave a gentle squeeze and looked into his father's face, seeing the aging process for maybe the first time. "I'll take you home."

"No need. My driver is waiting for me at the front."

Of course he was. "Let's get together for lunch sometime, then."

"I'll contact you."

That made Sam smile. Some things would never change. Well...maybe they would, but it would be in small increments.

As Carter made his way out of the door with a backhanded wave, some of the weight lifted from Sam's shoulders. All might not be right with his world, but at least it wasn't all wrong either. And he might need to learn to be content with that.

CHAPTER TEN

LUCY SLID INTO the conference room feeling a weird sense of déjà vu. This was how her entry into the facial-reanimation team had started. Only it hadn't carried the heartache that it did today. She hadn't seen Sam since the day he'd appeared in her department and asked for that flash drive. And he'd given no indication that he noticed anything different about her, other than that curt question about whether she found the whole situation amusing. She guessed her acting job had been a little too convincing.

But while she might've appeared fine on the outside, on the inside she was dealing with a pain that just would not quit. Had she felt this horrible after Matt had broken up with her?

She and Sam hadn't even been a couple. They'd slept together. One. Time.

So why was she having trouble sleeping and eating? But most of all why was she now considering giving up something she'd wanted so badly a month ago?

Because even the thought of seeing Sam, much less talking to him, caused a kind of anxiety she'd never experienced before. Todd had called her into his office and thanked her for all of the work on the protocol presentation and said it had been sent around to the rest of the team, who'd been unanimous in their approval of it.

Even talking about the project made her shrink away. She'd debated on not coming today. But this was the big Q&A that everyone had been looking forward to. And she was hoping for a sign that would send her in one direction or the other.

She found an empty seat and slid into it, noting that the panel was already in place on the podium, a microphone in front of each of the players, although one spot was empty. She swallowed, spotting Sam talking to one of the people at the front. He smiled at something the other man said, and it made her squirm.

She didn't think she could do this.

Lucy had been hoping her feelings would fade away, kind of in the same way they had when Matt had left. But these were still as strong as they'd been that day she discovered she loved Sam.

She still loved him. And she knew he was real

and authentic in a way that Matthew had not been. He hadn't tried to play games with her or vaguely say things that weren't true. He'd had no problem agreeing with her that sleeping together had been a mistake.

Of course, she'd been pretty blithe in the way she'd presented it. But her reasons for thinking it was a mistake were probably very different from his.

Sam turned around and started to come down the steps. As he reached the floor, his eyes met hers for a minute. He stopped and held her gaze steady for a minute before his lips thinned and he glanced away. The move wasn't a fluke. He was telling her in no uncertain terms where they stood.

And it was not on good ground.

She'd done okay holed up in her own department over the last week, except for that day he'd come down to see her. She was confident she could still work in the PT department. But Sam *was* the facial-reanimation department. He wasn't some minor player on the team. Everything revolved around him, and as such he would oversee every part of it. Which meant multiple conversations every time a new patient came through MMH's doors.

She'd actually gone to Human Resources and

asked if there was someone who could take her place on the team if it turned out she had to step down.

Melissa had pressed her, telling Lucy she could trust her with whatever she needed to say. Lucy had simply said some personal things had come up and she was rethinking her involvement. Her friend had told her to think long and hard about her decision, that opportunities like this didn't come along every day. She even offered to lighten her load in PT if that was the problem.

Lightening her load would only give her more time to think…to dread and probably avoid any interaction with Sam, which she knew meant she couldn't give the job what it needed. It needed someone who was there wholeheartedly for the patients no matter what conflicts she might have with any of the other team members. And there were no conflicts. Other than the one raging inside of her own heart.

To stay or to go. That was the question, and one she still couldn't answer.

What she needed right now was some air. Lucy glanced at her watch. She still had five more minutes until the event started. She grabbed a water bottle on her way through the door and unscrewed the cap, taking a long drink of the cool liquid as she headed to a nearby wall, leaning against it.

She needed to at least stay for this, no matter how she felt about Sam. She wanted to hear what these experts had to say, and there was a physical therapist listed as one of the speakers. There was a short bio on each person, but she really didn't recognize any of the names.

Leaning her head against the wall, she closed her eyes and took another drink, the cool liquid soothing her heated emotions in a way that helped, surprisingly.

"Hello." A voice to her left caught her attention, and her eyes opened to find a woman looking at her.

"Hi." There was something vaguely familiar about the person, and she stood there trying to figure out why.

"You're Lucy, aren't you?"

She peered closer. The woman knew her, and she tried to grasp where she knew her from. "I am. I know you, don't I?"

The woman was probably in her early thirties. When she smiled there was a slight crookedness to it that made Lucy tilt her head, and there was a slightly accented tone to her speech.

"You probably don't remember me. I looked a little different fifteen years ago."

Fifteen years ago. She hadn't even been a physical therapist at the time. She'd been studying to be...

Recognition gripped her and tears sprang to Lucy's eyes. She grabbed the woman in a hug and held her tight. "Oh, my God! I've worried about you all these years."

The woman hugged her back. "I've wanted to thank you all these years. I felt like you were the only one who really heard me back then."

It was the Moebius patient who'd been struggling so much. Lucy let go of her. "I don't even know your name."

"It's Becky Collins." She smiled. "Well, it is now. It was Becky Moore back then. I'm married, with three little ones."

"I'm so happy for you. You got your surgery, obviously."

"I did. More than one of them. It was a fight every step of the way, but I just remember you gripping my hand and telling me not to give up no matter what happened. I didn't. And here I am."

Becky looked at her for a long moment. "I came because I saw your name on the list of the team and asked to come along, although I had to shift some of my patients around."

"You're a doctor." Lucy breathed the word, unable to believe this was happening.

"I'm actually a physical therapist."

A ball of emotion lodged in her throat and wouldn't let go. Hers was the empty seat on the podium.

Becky touched her hand. "I'm so glad to know you'll be helping more people like me. I've dedicated my life to doing the same."

How could Lucy tell her that she'd been toying with dropping off the team? Her problems suddenly seemed so minor. Well, they weren't. But in the whole scope of things they were. MMH wasn't the only hospital that was building a program like this. There were other places out there doing this too. It was a growing field offering people a chance to be able to freely express their emotions through their facial muscles.

Like the ones she was currently suppressing? The ones that had her feeling she was slowly dying inside even as she kept on smiling on the outside. She didn't have to give up this dream. She just had to decide *where* she was going to do it.

"What's wrong?"

Becky was looking into her face, twin frown lines appearing.

God. It really was miraculous. She grabbed

Becky's hand. "I know you have to go inside and be on the panel, but can I talk to you later?"

"You can talk to me right now. You took the time to listen to me when I needed it the most—the least I can do is listen to you."

So even though they were basically strangers, Lucy felt an affinity with Becky that had her spilling out everything that had happened over the last month, how she'd slowly fallen in love with the new department's team leader and that she was thinking of resigning from her position.

"Did you tell him how you feel?"

Lucy shook her head. "No. I just keep smiling and trying to suppress my emotions."

"Hmmm. Just because you're *able* to smile doesn't mean you should."

She blinked. "I'm sorry?"

"I was so happy to have muscles that obeyed my mental commands that I sometimes pasted a smile on my face just because I could. It became a problem. One my husband had to talk to me about. So now I'm more careful." Becky paused. "How is he going to know it's bothering you if your face doesn't match what's inside?"

"But I can't just tell him."

Her brows went up slightly. "Why not? If you're thinking of stepping down anyway, what do you have to lose?"

"Maybe everything."

Becky hugged her. "And maybe you have everything to gain. Maybe he's fooled by your smile and doesn't think you care about him."

Lucy swallowed. "But what if it doesn't matter to him either way?"

"If I were you, I would want to know."

"Should I draw two circles?" She tried to make light of her problems by referring to their meeting all those years ago.

Becky shook her head. "No. Because no matter what happens in the first circle, life is still worth living. I found that out. Thanks to you. Even if I hadn't had my surgeries."

"Thank you. Thank you so much."

She nodded. "Ready to go back inside?"

"I'm ready."

Sam sat in his chair, a pain in his head that just wouldn't quit. He'd come down those stairs and glanced across the audience and seen Lucy. That was when it hit him. The pain. The pain in his head. The pain in his gut. And the pain in his chest. It had nothing to do with being sick or anything else. He'd caught Lucy at a time when she hadn't been smiling or laughing or joking about something, and he realized how much he missed all of those things.

This week without seeing her had been a strange one. It was like the joy of living had been sucked right out of him. At first he'd thought it had been just coming off the adrenaline rush from getting this Q&A organized and off the ground. But then when he saw Lucy, he knew exactly what it was, and it floored him. He was in love with the woman.

God, he didn't want to be and knew he didn't deserve someone like her and couldn't ask her to take a chance on him, but it had hurt to look away. And then when he'd chanced to glance back there again, she'd been gone. And he wanted nothing more than to run out that door and find her. But of course he couldn't. And he shouldn't.

She was doing just fine without him—she'd made that very clear the last time they'd spoken. So he should just let things rest the way they were.

But how was he going to work with her?

He didn't know, and that was something he'd have to sort through later. There would be a time and place for all of that. But it wasn't now.

After an hour and a half, there were finally no more questions. Todd went up to the front and stood at the microphone. "Our guest panel has been kind enough to offer to stay afterward for a while and answer any questions you may not have wanted to ask in an open forum, but one member of the panel has asked to say something to all of you."

A woman came to the microphone and stood with Todd. She looked a little uncomfortable standing in front of everyone, but she smiled.

"My name is Becky, and I have Moebius syndrome."

Sam's gaze sharpened. She'd been on the panel and had answered questions just like the other members of the team, and he hadn't noticed anything specifically different about her.

She went on. "I can't tell you how important the facial-reanimation field is, but you all feel it, or you wouldn't be here. I have a special friend here who gave me hope at a time when I felt I had none. You'll never know how happy I am to see her on this team and to see her here today. I hope she'll never doubt her importance to this field, no matter where she may find herself. Thanks to all of you."

She then went back to her seat.

Sam's gaze jerked back to where Lucy was sitting and saw tears streaming down her face, and he knew in a moment who that woman was. But why had she said *no matter where she may find herself*? Was Lucy thinking of leaving MMH? Surely not.

Hell, he surely didn't want to be the reason for that—although she'd seemed fine when he'd talked to her, so he might have misconstrued the woman's words. But the thought of never seeing Lucy again? The pain in his midsection grew in intensity. He'd only felt relief after he and Priscilla broke up. And he hadn't missed her since being back in the States. But Lucy?

That was another story. He already missed her, even though they worked in the same building.

So what was he going to do about it? He wasn't sure, but he'd better figure it out pretty damned quick.

Lucy was gone. He'd finished saying farewell to the last of the visiting experts and had gone and personally had a word with Becky, thanking her for her words and for being willing to put herself out there for others who needed the same life-changing surgeries. She'd smiled. "I feel like I already know you. But thanks for your kind words."

With that she was gone. She felt like she already knew him?

Had she spoken with Lucy and been told that she was thinking of going somewhere else?

When he'd looked for her, the room was empty and she was nowhere to be seen. Sam glanced at his phone, and the screen was blank. No texts. So she hadn't tried to reach him. Maybe she was down in her department. If so, he needed to find her and tell her the truth. If she didn't feel the same and thought they couldn't work together, he would understand. But why should she be the one to leave a place she'd worked for her entire career? If anyone should go, it should be him.

And he was going to make that clear.

With that in mind he headed out the door and started in the direction of the elevator until something to his left caught his eye. He glanced over there and saw Lucy, standing there all by herself.

Okay, there she was. Let's see if he could do what he said he was going to do. He went over. "Can I talk to you for a few minutes?"

"Yes. I was just waiting for you, actually."

So she *was* leaving. She'd just stayed here tell him.

"Let's go to my office."

She shook her head. "I'd rather go to that quiet little waiting room just down the hall from there. There's rarely anyone there."

"Okay." That didn't bode well for whatever it was she wanted to say.

The conference room was housed on the same floor as the plastic-surgery wing, so they went just around the corner and found the area she was talking about.

She led the way and went to the far back corner and sat down. He joined her, careful not to touch her. His heart ached in a way he'd never known. But he had to do this now, or he'd always regret it.

"Are you thinking of leaving MMH?"

Lucy nodded, and none of her customary exuberance was on display at the moment. "I actually thought about stepping down from the team, but then I saw Becky in the hallway and she convinced me that I should rethink that. That if things couldn't work out here, and if I really cared about the facial-reanimation field, I should find another place where I can plug in. And I really do care."

"Why? Why do you want to leave?"

"Can't you guess?" She gazed into his eyes, and he saw nothing but Lucy. The Lucy he'd come to know.

"Is it because we slept together?"

"No. It's because of what I realized after it happened."

He took a deep breath. "And what was that?"

"That I'd fallen in love with you and that it was going to be hell to work on a team where I saw you each and every day." Her eyes held steady.

"But down in your treatment room you seemed so happy and even said—"

"I was lying. And Becky helped me to see that when my facial expressions don't match what I'm feeling inside, it means I'm not being truthful to myself or to the person I'm addressing. I need to learn the importance of being authentic."

"Well, then I've been lying too. Only I just realized it during the Q&A."

"And what were you lying about?"

Now she was frowning. And it made him smile. "I kept telling myself that these feelings I had for you would go away even when deep down I knew they wouldn't. I love you. And when your friend Becky stood up and hinted that you might be leaving, my world might as well have imploded. I don't want you to leave, Lucy. I want you to stay. And work with me. And be beside me always. In good times and bad."

"But you said you didn't want to be with anyone."

"At that time, I didn't. Because of my upbringing. Because of Priscilla. Because of the lies I told myself all along the way. I didn't believe I could be fully engaged with anyone emotionally. But our night together…let's just say it made me rethink that. Not just physically. But yes, emotionally. I've never felt more in tune with another human being than I do when I'm with you. And it wasn't just that night. It was when I saw you with Devon. When we walked in the park and talked about things that were more than just superficial." He shrugged. "When I told you about my arrest. I love you. That's the only explanation. And if you can help me get past the times when I have problems being like you said… authentic, or at least hold me accountable, I'd like to try to make this work."

"Are you serious?"

He smiled. "About holding me accountable or trying to make this work? Because I'm very serious about both of those things."

"Then, yes, Sam, to both." She took his hand. "I sat in that conference room thinking I couldn't go through with being on the team, and then I saw Becky in the hallway. She convinced me to come talk to you and tell you the truth."

"She didn't tell me exactly that same thing, but she convinced me to do the same."

Lucy sighed. "She's a special lady."

"Yes, she is." Sam leaned down and kissed her on the mouth. "I love you, Luce."

"I love you too." She smiled. "*Dios*. It's good to smile and have it feel real."

"It's good to see you smile and know it's real." He stood and held out his hand. "Shall we?"

She took his hand and let him pull her out of the chair. Then with his arm around her waist, they walked out into the corridor. "What are people going to think if they see us like this?"

"Who cares? They can either be happy for us, or they can go to—"

She put her hand over his mouth to stop the word before it came out. "Let's just hope they're happy for us in the same way that I'm happy for us."

Sam dropped a kiss onto her head. "I am too."

A coy smile appeared on her face, and she glanced up at him. "So is that extra spot in front of your apartment only available on street-sweeper days?"

A laugh bubbled from his chest that felt good and healing and right. "It's available anytime you want it to be. And I'm hoping it's every single night."

"Oh, mister, you may regret saying that."

"Never. I'll never regret anything when it comes to you."

And they walked down the hallway smiling at anyone who happened to look their way, knowing they were heading into a future that would make a difference. Not just for them, but for lots of other people who would walk the halls of MMH in search of answers and hopefully find what they were looking for.

EPILOGUE

SAM AND LUCY stood at the front with only their closest friends and relatives gathered around them. Sam had not been interested in big festivities—he wanted this to be done like he'd lived most of his life: simply. The fact that Lucy had been the one to bring it up first had confirmed for the millionth time that he could do this emotional journey. He'd just needed the right partner by his side.

Surprisingly his parents had not argued for a huge elaborate wedding. Maybe they'd learned their lesson from what happened with Logan and Harper. But he had to say grandparenthood looked good on both of his parents. They doted on his brother's baby girl, and Lily, in turn, seemed to adore them.

His dad had softened in ways that were unimaginable. His and Sam's relationship would never be perfect—they wanted different things out of life—but for the most part they had come to an understanding. And Sam had told him he loved him and had meant it.

The officiant repeated words that Sam had heard so many times before at other people's weddings, but this time each syllable became an oath that he vowed to keep. He loved Lucy more today than he had eight months ago at their first meeting. And when they'd started the Pediatric Microsurgery and Facial-Reanimation Department, they never could have imagined how successful it would come to be. They'd already performed and done physical therapy on ten kids, all of them with hopeful outcomes.

But as successful as it was, he and Lucy had carved out a month of time away from the hospital to go to Paraguay and spend time learning about Lucy's heritage. And where she could curse in Spanish without heads turning in her direction.

She was beautiful. Both inside and out, and he was so, so lucky to be able to share this life with her.

Becky was standing beside her as her maid of honor, along with Lucy's sister, Bella. Lucy and Becky had reconnected in a way that went beyond friendship, and she'd become like family, along with her kids and husband. They visited whenever they could.

The month away would also give them time to start trying to have a family of their own away from the stressors of the hospital and craziness of life. They could lounge around and enjoy each other and revel in the chance they'd been given.

"Repeat after me." The man glanced at Sam and then back again when Sam couldn't stop the smile that spread across his face. He'd decided that he'd fallen in love long before he realized he was in love. It was the time Lucy had worn those parrot scrubs with its motto scrawled across them and he'd decided he needed to make that motto his own.

"Sorry," Sam said. "Inside joke."

When he glanced at Lucy, she was grinning too. He was probably lucky she hadn't stuck a puppet onto his hand and asked him to do his vows in animal voices. But if she'd asked, he would have done it. Anything for this woman.

They each repeated what the minister recited, and Sam's eyes never left his bride's. When he finally told them they could kiss each other, he'd swung her up into his arms and kissed her in tiny little touches that he hoped paved the way for some longer and sexier kisses later. But first they had the reception to get to.

Like the ceremony, it would be held at the hospital in its little courtyard that had been reserved for just this moment.

He carried her past family and friends and finally set her down just outside of the small chapel. "I love you, Lucy Galeano-Grant."

"I love you too, Sam. And I can't wait to introduce you to…" She pulled a plastic strip from somewhere inside her wedding dress and held it up to him.

He glanced at it, baffled, before realizing what it was. "What? Already?"

"Yep. We can go on our honeymoon without worrying about at least one thing."

He put his hand on her belly and whispered, "Welcome to our family, little one. Get ready for a wild ride."

"Sam!"

"What?" He gave her a naughty grin. "I was talking about life, not…"

She laughed, and that sound carried with Sam as they went out into the courtyard…as they headed for the table with their wedding cake… and as they headed into their future together.

* * * * *

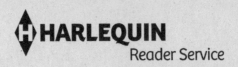

HARLEQUIN
Reader Service

Enjoyed your book?

Try the perfect subscription for Romance readers and get more great books like this delivered right to your door.

See why over 10+ million readers have tried Harlequin Reader Service.

Start with a Free Welcome Collection with free books and a gift—valued over $20.

Choose any series in print or ebook.
See website for details and order today:

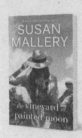 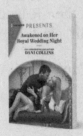 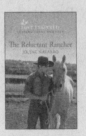 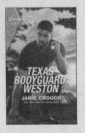

TryReaderService.com/subscriptions